SUCCESSFUL PRACTITIONERS
IN
CANINE
REHABILITATION & PHYSIOTHERAPY

D1739255

SUCCESSFUL PRACTITIONERS

IN
CANINE
REHABILITATION
& PHYSIOTHERAPY

Laurie Edge-Hughes

First Printing 2014

ISBN: 978-0-9812431-6-0

Publisher:

Four Leg Rehab Inc
PO Box 1581,
Cochrane, AB
T4C 1B5 Canada
www.FourLeg.com
Your place for online canine rehab education!

Cover photo (Laurie Edge-Hughes & Jasper Campos) credit to:
Janet Pliszka,
Visual Hues Photography

Inside photo (Vader Nichols Zoller) credit to:
Mike Kehn,
M Kehn Photography

Book cover and interior design by Jean Boles
http://jeanboles.elance.com

Contents

Contributors are listed alphabetically by their first name

Introduction

Many people have asked me how the idea came for this book. Really, the answer is simple. Since I've been "around" for so long in the animal rehab field, I have had a chance to meet (and stay in contact with, or semi-regularly bump into) others in the field. Most of us struggled at some point to see our practice take off, and within each of our stories comes threads of wisdom. Wisdom that has been hard earned. We've tried things; we've sometimes failed; we've sometimes succeeded, and we've grown as practitioners and business people along the way. And our stories are useful, both as a learning tool for others, but also as a record of the collective history of the field of animal rehab/physiotherapy. My hope for this book is that it helps and inspires those new to the field and those already in the field who may be looking for new ideas, solutions or validation of their current path and/or style of practice. As well, I hope that we can move forwards together to realize the dreams and visions that practitioners in this field see for the practice of animal rehab.

How did this book take shape? Well, as I said previously, I've been around for a while in this field, and I've met many a practitioner in my day. So I first created a list of people I knew who had been practicing in the field for a while, or who had unique stories and perspectives that I knew about. I then created a list of questions that I thought would give reader insights into a) how people started, b) how they currently practice, c) how they market, d) their advice for others, and e) a few other questions that I thought would be useful to know. Then I sent the surveys and invitations to participate out to my list of practitioners... followed by a reminder (or two). So at this point, if you are reading this and thinking, "Hey, I've known Laurie for years, and I didn't get a survey," I'd put money on it that you are one of the ones that didn't respond—perhaps you need to check your junk folder more often! Not to publicly chastise anyone, but there are some people whose stories, I would have loved to have shared, who either didn't get back to me, or who told me at the time that they were too busy. So the group of professionals contained within these pages is not an exhaustive list of successful canine re-hab/physio practitioners… but they are the ones who got their butts in gear to help me complete this project!

Now I also have to tell you that this book took far longer to compile than I originally thought it would! My apologies to the participants who have been eagerly awaiting its arrival for over a year now! Which also means that the information contained within is relevant to the time at which each person completed the questionnaire: A snapshot in time, if you will.

Without further ado, I hope you find enjoyment, enlightenment, or energy when you read the stories.

Cheers to your success in Practice!
Laurie Edge-Hughes,
BScPT, MAnimSt (Animal Physio), CAFCI, CCRT
Cochrane, Alberta, Canada 2013

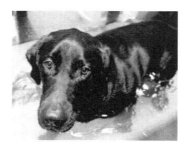

**'Vader' enjoying an underwater treadmill session
At The Canine Fitness Centre in Calgary.**

Amie Lamoreaux Hesbach,

MSPT, DPT(c), CCRP, CCRT
Massachusetts Veterinary Referral Hospital,
Intown Veterinary Group (IVG))
Woburn, MA, USA
www.ivghospitals.com
Ph: 781.932.5802
E-mail: ahesbach@ivghospitals.com / forpawsrehab@gmail.com

How did it all begin for you, Amie?

Hmmm... So I was the typical kid who wanted to be a veterinarian, along with an airline stewardess (what they USED to call them), and a ballerina, etc. etc. I had a well-meaning aunt tell me that she couldn't be a veterinarian because she couldn't put dogs and cats to sleep. That was all it took to make me drop that idea! My mom was a nurse, and in her day, the only appropriate jobs for women were secretary (also what they USED to call them), nurse, or teacher. So I went the route of physical therapy, close to nursing but not so gory (until I saw that we did wound care! But it was too late—I was in school by then). I steered my learning path through undergrad, PT school, and landed my first job.

Settling in, my boyfriend (soon to be husband) bought a house, and we agreed that he needed a dog. Enter Kate, my now 14-year-old border collie. Along the way, we dog sat a friend's Chesapeake Bay retriever, Orville. He had had a rough life and had horrible back posture. He was so sway-backed that his belly was lower to the ground than I thought acceptable. I tried some of my NDT [Neurodevelopmental Technique] tricks and found, wow, this stuff really did work. Neuromuscular re-education on DOGS!

Soon afterwards, I moved to California to do my PNF [Proprio-ceptive Neuromuscular Facilitation] residency. I soooo missed my dog, and I remember going to Chrissy Field in San Francisco just to watch the dogs. I bought a Canine Orthopaedics book from Barnes & Noble (it wasn't of great caliber, however). But I started to study a little from that point. I returned to Maryland (now engaged) and talked to Kate's DVM about these crazy courses that I kept seeing (from the American Physical Therapy Association) on Canine Rehabilitation. He hooked me up with two veterinary surgeons who were LOOKING for a PT and the rest was history!

Where do you practice now?
I work out of a veterinary referral hospital. The service sees 10 – 12 cases per day (so about 50 – 72 patients per week) over a five to six day workweek. We are staffed with one Physical Therapist (PT) full time; one PT (as able/needed); one part-time DVM; two rehab aides, and the medical director is a DVM, CCRP, DACVS. The caseload is comprised of 60% postsurgical orthopaedics, 20% neurological, 10% orthopaedic (non-surgical), and 10% other (geriatrics, internal medicine, trauma, pneumonia, inpa-tients).

Generally, cases are referred to the rehab department from in-ternal sources (surgery, neuro, internal medicine, ICU/Emergency, or Cardiovascular) or externally from client and general practice DVMs. Additionally, we receive external refer-rals from Tufts or Angell (another referral center in Boston). I evaluate, treat, and delegate to techs/aides as appropriate. We charge based on both time and/or modality. We charge for un-derwater treadmill and laser differently than the 'rehab/PT' ses-sions. We do also offer packaged rates.

Advertising?

We do have a marketing gal, but she's pretty overwhelmed! We have brochures, a website, do e-blasts, create newsletters, purchase advertisements, sponsor events (e.g. fairs, gay-pride parade, etc.), and word of mouth, of course. I'm not sure what my favorite would be, and I'm not really able to provide further feedback on what has been the best or worst.

Tell us about your strengths and how you maintain or improve upon your skills...

I tend to focus on meeting the "client's" goal to get them invested in their pet's health and recovery. I also focus on the positive and can offer a service to them that the pet might not have had before (PT by a PT, not a DVM or tech). All of my training, education, and experience as a PT are my greatest assets. THAT cannot be replicated in any certification course or internship. My PNF residency changed me as a PT practitioner.

To keep sharp, I'm currently working on my tDPT [transitional Doctorate in Physical Therapy]. I spend time studying/reading veterinary and PT literature and going to rounds at our hospital. I also have a close network of PT colleagues that I use as a sounding board for difficult cases. I attend continuing education courses (human PT) to gain new skills. So my goals are to finish my tDPT, complete certification in "Graston technique," take more manual therapy courses and maybe take a vacation!

I struggle with balancing my focus on my professional development, my family, and the needs of my clients, patients, and referral sources.

Comment on educational opportunities in the field…

They're lacking and need improvement. There also needs to be more research/publications on manual therapies and PT-focused interventions. We need MORE! Period. And we're all busy—bogged down by our own political/legislative issues, etc.

Why do you think that some struggle to make an animal rehab practice successful?

I think some practitioners/clinics fail because it can be difficult to demonstrate the value of the service to prospective clients. Rehab can be costly for the client; it's labor intensive, and it is expensive to purchase all of the equipment and "bells and whistles."

There's also no "standard of practice."

If I were to start over, I might have maintained more autonomy as a practitioner, and not married myself to one practice when I was practicing in Maryland. I might also have maintained a mobile business, relying more on my hands and brain than the toys (bells and whistles) that attract so much attention.

The future of animal rehab from your point of view?

In the future, DVMs will continue to "do rehab," but it will be very different than the practice or rehab by PTs. I see these two groups diverging even more in their practice. PTs need to continue to emphasize their strengths to referral sources and clients, as we understand movement and kinematics better than other professionals. Also, we can offer something to the client as well. I feel that we animal rehab PTs can offer so much to our clients in education and injury prevention.

I'd like to see us all get along. I'd like to see the PT practice as we do best—managing the patients' movement deficits. I'd like to see the DVM focus more on medical-rehab management and for the technician to be doing the technical work.

Your advice...

Be a sponge. Build experience as a PT first then get your hands wet/furry with animal patients. Find a mentor (or two or three).

Amy Kramer,

PT, DPT, CCRT
California Animal Rehabilitation
Santa Monica, California
www.CalAnimalRehab.com
310-998-CARE (2273)
AKramer@CalAnimalRehab.com

In the beginning...

My own dog, "Lucy," a six-year-old Rottweiler, had TPLO surgery, and afterward the surgeon was thrilled that she was weight-bearing. However, I wasn't thrilled because she lacked the ROM she needed to get herself through the dog door. When I asked the surgeon what I could do, his response was "you're a physical therapist; you should be able to help her." Now had he mentioned a rehab facility that I could take her to, it would have been perfect. However, since no one was doing anything other than swim therapy in Los Angeles, the thought crossed my mind, "Why isn't anyone doing rehab on pets?" On my way home I picked up a dog anatomy book, and to my surprise, I found that the anatomy was pretty similar to humans. My Lucy turned out to be a perfect patient and tolerated soft tissue work, joint mobilizations and stretching, and within two weeks she had full ROM and went through the dog door just like before! At that moment I found my calling!

Funny how when I was a kid I wanted to be a vet, and so now I get to combine my two loves for the perfect career fit. I finished my canine rehab certification in 2005, and in 2007, I partnered with a veterinarian to open California Animal Rehab (CARE).

Tell us about CARE

We are in a rehab specialty clinic and all we do is rehab, including acupuncture, underwater treadmill, etc. We have both veterinarians and physical therapists all certified in rehabilitation, seeing the pet each visit. On any given day there are two full-time PTs and two full-time vets on staff. We also have eight technicians working daily, as well, to facilitate the PTs and vets. Our clinic sees about 250 pets per week and is open six days a week (40 – 50 pets/day). Approximately 50% of our caseload is ortho, 40% is neuro, and 10% is fitness/conditioning. In general, about 70% of our pets would be considered geriatric.

What does rehab at CARE look like for a patient?

The pet first comes to the clinic for the initial consultation where the rehab program is recommended. Depending on the pet's problems and needs, the therapy sessions will either be a 30-minute acupuncture visit followed by 30 minutes with a rehab assistant and physical therapist, or 30 minutes with a rehab assistant and physical therapist and 30 minutes for underwater treadmill. This does not mean that they are in the UWTM for 30 minutes! We have set protocols for time, speed, etc. based on the pet's problems (i.e. de-conditioned, ataxic, degenerative, etc.) Regardless of whether the owner selected a packaged set of sessions or is paying per session, the pet does rehab for four weeks and then we re-evaluate in order to modify the program as needed.

Initial consults at CARE are conducted with the rehab DVM, which lasts two hours. At that time it is determined what type of "program" the pet would most benefit from. The majority of our "ortho" cases select a twice-a-week package. This includes the initial consult, 15 (1-hour) therapy sessions, a re-evaluation (at 4 weeks) and a final evaluation (at 8 weeks). At each of the evaluations we compare the objective findings and measurements to those found at the initial evaluation. Most of the neurologic cases opt to come three times a week or more. Each of the packages has a set price. If they purchase a package, they receive a discount. We also allow clients to "pay as they go," but ultimately, we charge by the visit not the modality.

Tell us about your referrals and how you advertise?
We have a large referral base from local surgeons and general practitioners. We tend to see plenty of self-referrals as well from clients that find our website via various search engines. Lastly, "word of mouth" is huge, and our happy clients eagerly refer us to their friends.

We spend a lot of time marketing to the local DVM community through lunch talks, intern education, veterinary association presentations, and distribution of our marketing materials (i.e., flyers/brochures and post-surgical handouts). We take out ads in certain magazines and find other venues, magazines, television ads, and radio spots that will assist in getting our name out in front of the public. As well, we send out quarterly or bi-annual newsletters, and we have a constantly updated and changing website and Facebook page. Lastly, we take pictures and videos of our patients doing therapy and we e-mail those to each client with our logo and website listed, and they, in turn, forward those to their friends and it goes viral!

What has been your greatest strength?
I truly believe that the reason that we are successful both personally and as a clinic, is the fact that we combine the two professions by having physical therapists and veterinarians working together on each case. We have an understanding and a respect for each other and acknowledge and appreciate what the other

profession brings to the table. I think it gives us the ability to offer the pet the best outcomes in rehabilitation.

When I first had the idea to open a rehab clinic, my first step was
to find a DVM who shared my views and could help the practice
thrive and offer services that I, as a PT, would not have been able
to offer (i.e., acupuncture, nutrition counseling, supplement and
general animal medical knowledge that is key when treating a
pet.) I wouldn't have done anything different, as it has turned out
exactly as I had hoped.

Why do you think that some rehab facilities/departments fail?

I have always felt that marketing the right way is extremely important. We spend a lot of time and money on marketing, and it
truly pays off. I also feel that it is important not to step on the
toes of those you would like to refer to you. In other words, we
do not do anything that a general practice DVM or surgeon
would do, as we have no intentions of take away any of their
business. We want to be an adjunct to their services and offer
complementary services to help their clients. I have always felt
that a freestanding rehab specialty clinic will always do better
than a rehab clinic within a surgical center, because being inside
a surgical hospital or general practice you are likely to limit the
number of outside referrals you will get. For example, a surgeon
will hesitate or refrain from sending their client to another surgical facility just for rehab for fear that they will lose their client
to the facility that "has it all under one roof." Lastly, I think that
DVM's often think that by adding an underwater treadmill
(UWTM) in a small room means that they offer "rehab." When in
fact, a true rehab practitioner knows that, A) not all pets are
good candidates for UWTM, B) there is a lot more to rehab than
the UWTM, and C) to offer rehab correctly you need to have pro-

fessionals that understand and are certified in rehab working with the pets (i.e. a tech running an UWTM is not rehab).

What are the struggles of rehab practice and what would advise would you give to new practitioners?

I think the biggest challenge has been convincing the surgeons and general practice DVM's that there are other options to surgery and drugs, and that rehab has a valuable place in pet healthcare and should be a first consideration, not an afterthought. I would like rehab to be the FIRST choice versus the second or last chance. I would like rehab to be like it is in the human world, where the doctors say, "let's try rehab first, and if that doesn't work then we can consider surgery." Surgery will always be an option, but you will never know if rehab would have worked if you do surgery first! I also wish to see rehab become mainstream, such that any pet that has a surgical procedure goes to rehab immediately—not wait until the pet doesn't get better after several months and then gets referred to rehab.

Getting started in this field requires marketing, marketing, and more marketing! Educate the DVM's you expect to refer to you; make sure they understand that rehab is NOT doggy daycare or just swimming. Educate them that their patients will look better with rehab than without it, and then prove it to them!

What is your next step?

Currently we are looking to expand our space, as we have outgrown our current facility. We are looking at expanding our services as well to include fitness and wellness. We learned a lot from building the first facility, and we look forward to making a better more efficient facility in the future.

Ann Essner,

BSc Physical Therapy, RPT, RPT Veterinary Medicine
Gefle Hund & Kattpraktik (www.geflehundokattpraktik.se)
+46 26 10 63 10
E-mail: ann@geflehundokattpraktik.se
VETFYSIO (www.vetfysio.com) +46 70 692 75 62
E-mail: ann.essner@bredband.net
Gävle, Sweden

When did you start, Ann? And what does it mean "RPT Veterinary Medicine"?

I started practicing canine physiotherapy on a regular basis in 2002, starting at one day a week. (*The RPT Veterinary Medicine was approved by the Swedish Board of Agriculture to allow physiotherapists to practice within veterinary medicine with the same supervising authority as registered vets and registered vet nurses in Sweden.*)

Getting started

I was involved in LSVET (Swedish Association of Registered Physiotherapists within Veterinary Medicine—www.lsvet.se) from the very beginning. We formed the organization in 1994. In 1999, the Swedish University of Agricultural Sciences started a course in veterinary medicine for physiotherapists, which I had the opportunity to take. Before the course was finished in 2003, I made contact with a highly skilled veterinary orthopedic surgeon. He was looking for collaboration within the field of physical rehabilitation in veterinary medicine. Professor DVM Håkan Kasström became a very important mentor to me.

Ann's canine rehab practice(s)

I am employed as a physical therapist at a veterinary clinic full-time (40 hours a week). There are seven vets and eleven vet nurses at the main clinic, and we also have a small branch clinic in a nearby town. The clinic operates the physio/rehab department with one physiotherapist and one vet nurse. It is most important in that everyone in the clinic views physiotherapy as an important part of the clinic.

Gefle Hund & Kattpraktik sees 19,000 patients a year. (The small branch clinic is not included in this number.) I offer 10-15 bookable visits a day in my schedule, which accounts for approximately 50 or more patient visits per week. 80% of the caseload is ortho or neuro rehab; 15% is fitness; 5% is strictly geriatric (but this group also fits within the ortho and neuro group as well). For physiotherapy services, we have a separate room where the water treadmill is kept and in the adjacent room is a fully equipped vet clinic room. I have close access to all of my measurement tools, TENS, kinesiotape and other PT stuff. The UWTM room has its own entrance and exit to be used if necessary.

Clients pay for services based on time, we sometimes offer a pre-paid package (i.e. 5-10 visits), and in some cases insurance companies pay part of the cost for clients. Personally, I don't like pre-paid package. I want the client to utilize as many visits as needed. This might be only one visit for some of the dogs or cats, but more often repeated visits are necessary. It is difficult to determine how many visits will be required at the beginning when the clients are buying the packages. Although, I have experienced that clients sometimes like pre-paid packages. So, this strategy might be a good sales trick.

How do you advertise and get referrals?

Most of our referrals come from the vets at our clinic or other veterinary referral centers. We do almost no advertising at all. It is mostly word of mouth!

I try to work with a "happy face" and let my clients be aware of that I love what I am doing. I use an ethical and moral approach, where I let my clients know what I do and what they may expect if they do their part in the rehab process (i.e. the home program and following advice). I try to be honest with my clients and together with my vets, deliver a professional diagnosis and prognosis in regards the treatment(s) we may offer. Sometimes it is to gently recommend to euthanize the dog or cat. When this happens, the clients seem to appreciate this and will return for care when needed for their other pets.

So far I have had many successes, and I am afraid that I might begin to experience clients that expect too much! When it comes to my job, I am still living my dream and I have not compromised my ethical or moral beliefs. With years of experience and continuing education, I hope I will survive!

Ann's strengths as a canine physiotherapist

I am a touch hyperactive and I like to stay busy. I look at the long-term, and I try to treat four-legged and two-legged patients in a way that makes them willing to come back. Even if it means that I recommend euthanizing a dog for an ethical reason, I know that that dog owner would come back if he or she needed my help in the future.

I also have training in some veterinary nursing skills. For example, I have training and legislated approval to inject medication subcutaneously and intramuscular. This means I can give dogs "Cartrophen Vet" injections and the like.

I am also curious by nature, which makes the opportunity of life-long learning in our profession as physiotherapists perfect for me. I maintain and upgrade my skills via international contacts, networking, and educational opportunities, and I have a few mentors within human and veterinary medicine. Continuing education in canine physiotherapy is lacking in my country. Hopefully, it is getting better.

Why do you think that some animal physiotherapy practitioners or facilities fail?

One reason for failure is if the facility doesn't employ a team-approach in regards to rehabilitation. I have been in such a situation before. The "work culture" and "how to apply and develop new thinking" is very different from place to place. Based on my experience, I have come to believe that it is not possible to practice rehabilitation and physical therapy on your own or in a small group of people at a small animal hospital where you are not supported. I eventually realized that I couldn't continue in an unsupportive model, and I left to work full-time with my current employer.

Ann's current goals, view of the future, and lessons learned

I plan to stay with my current employer and I will finish my master's degree. I am just about to prepare the thesis (the subject pertains to dogs, of course). I don't know my final results yet, and I'm curious to see how it turns out!

I would like to see animal physical therapy become part of rehabilitation medicine and not alternative medicine—worldwide!

It has been a long journey and I have learned a lot, both professionally and about myself. I don't regret anything I've done. I keep thinking that later on, the only things I will regret are those that I didn't do.

Advice from Ann

In the beginning your hobby will be your work, which means you need to take a serious interest in canine physiotherapy and improve your knowledge of animals. Start working side by side with your vets.

Ansi VanderWalt,

MSc Physiotherapy
EquiBalance Studio cc & Physiotherapy Solutions
Johannesburg, South Africa
www.equibalance.co.za & www.physiotherapysolutions.co.za
E-mail: ansi@equibalance.co.za

In the beginning...

I realized that physiotherapy on animals was what I wanted to do when I was about 16. The hardest part was trying to learn how one does this! I was accepted into the physiotherapy degree program at the University of Pretoria, and early on I started hanging around the veterinary faculty, wondering how the techniques and skills I was learning could be applied to the animals. Fortunately, the faculty was tolerant! They allowed me to try things on some of the patients, and I ended up doing a very nice case study on the treatment of cranial tibial tendinitis in a horse. I became involved in the Animal Physiotherapy Group as a student representative.

Luckily, I was able to secure my first job in a practice where one of the partners treated animals as well, and from the start I worked half day on people and half day on animals.

Ansi's practice

I own a private practice that focuses mostly on the treatment of small animals, but we do also treat horses and human patients. It is a true multispecies practice!

I see about 75 cases a week: 50% ortho; 40% neuro; 10% other (arthritis management, weights loss, and fitness). Onsite, we have one veterinary nurse, two aides and me. We charge per booking type; for example, water treadmill, physiotherapy (hands-on treatment), or group rehabilitation. If we do two different treatment types (e.g. hands-on and treadmill), we charge the second type at 50% discount. Consumables such as tape or bandages are extra.

As much as we would prefer primarily veterinary referrals, the bulk of our patients learn of our services by word-of-mouth referral. As the physiotherapist, I first assess every patient before a treatment plan is compiled. The treatment plan will differ from patient to patient. When the client arrives for therapy, the staff member allocated to the patient will begin with the pre-planned treatment, but the physiotherapist (or the vet nurse in simpler cases, such as weight loss) supervises all treatments, and treatment may be changed during the session if the supervisor feels that patient goals are not being achieved.

Advertising?

We have some advertising material in magazines and other publications, but while I believe that this is important for building brand awareness, it is not the best way to increase sales. People need to make a personal connection, either with you as a professional or via an acquaintance or veterinary professional.

Having a presence at events has proven to be very successful, provided it is done in a certain way. We offer free "sports massages or relaxation massages" for a donation to charity. Our only requirement is the animal owner's contact details and the form allows them to tick whether they want to receive the free newsletter or not. This way we can build rapport with them, they can ask questions, and we also build our database. The other important thing is to continually build on the relationships with the vets that refer to you, and always have marketing material available in the clinics!

What we have also started in South Africa are inter-professional journal clubs. We invite physios and vets to come together and compare literature on the treatment of specific conditions (e.g. sacroiliac joints in humans, horses and dogs).

Ansi's strengths and weaknesses
I feel that I have the ability to apply new knowledge and technologies from the human field to the treatment and rehabilitation of animals in a very practical way. I spend a lot of time with clients explaining injuries or pathological processes and subsequent expectation management. I feel it is very important to provide individually structured rehabilitation protocols—not recipes—and lastly, I stay closely involved with each case as much as possible, even when I am not directly treating the patient. I think all of these things have helped to make my practice successful.

I struggled with business management! We physios need to learn MUCH more about business. I learnt through mistakes—not advisable! I would suggest learning about business first— physiotherapists can already the physio-side of this area of practice!

Why do you think that some animal physiotherapy practitioners or facilities fail?
I think they don't realize at the outset how difficult it is going to be to marry the concept of animal physiotherapy (which seems like a good idea), with the realities of economic factors, practical application, education, and business management. This is espe-

cially true in an area of expertise (animal physiotherapy) where training is variable at best, evidence is poor, and competition for the resources available to spend on pets is limited.

Thoughts about education and how Ansi stays current

I think that educational opportunities in this field are severely lacking, but I do think that any educational programme based primarily on physical attendance by the delegate is doomed to fail. This method is too expensive, and because of the limited pool of experts in the field, it is too reliant on the input of too few to be sustainable. Any educational programme that wants to survive will have to utilize technology to survive.

I keep current primarily by self-studying. I also learn a tremendous amount from human courses where the theoretical bases of treatment techniques are explained. I find that the interaction and discussions with colleagues, like the journal clubs, is a very valuable tool for my learning as well. My next goal would be to do my PhD. I've just been too scared to start!

Dreams for the future of animal physiotherapy

Animal physiotherapy must become a more evidence-based profession. We need to conduct more research and more case studies. There are few advanced animal therapy courses, because there is little advanced knowledge on animal functional anatomy (e.g. the stability of the stifle joint). Compared to the human field, we are teaching more and more people to massage or apply TENS, but too few people are advancing knowledge. This makes the profession bottom-heavy. Certification courses are good to ensure safe practice but do not contribute to the evidence.

Any other advice?

You need to build relationships. Don't assume that just because you know you can add value, that other professionals know this as well. Also make sure your business model does not make other professionals feel threatened; you will need these people, even other physiotherapy practitioners, to support you.

And as an aside, clicker-training and cognitive behavioural therapy for dogs are VERY valuable and underutilized tools in rehabilitation!

Barbara Bockstahler,

DVM, CCRT, PhD,
Specialist veterinarian in physiotherapy & rehabilitation
University of Veterinary Medicine Vienna (Vetmeduni Vienna)
Vienna, Austria
http://www.vetmeduni.ac.at/tierspital/kliniken/kleintiere/klei
ntierchirurgie/physiotherapie/
E-mail: Barbara.bockstahler@vetmeduni.ac.at

Getting started

After my studies at the Vetmeduni, I went into private practice for some years. During this time, I started with an education in acupuncture. In 1999, the head of the clinic for internal medicine asked me if I would be interested in working at the university to build up a service for physiotherapy and acupuncture. (This service was started at the university around one year beforehand, but the governing position was now vacant.) So I started on this new career path, and the number of patients grew constantly. Internal medicine housed the physiotherapy and acupuncture service for about one year, but then it was transferred to the clinic for surgery, mainly because at the time the surgeons referred most of the patients. I can remember that our first room for physiotherapy was very small, and we worked only with our hands and acupuncture needles. Over time we were able to buy more equipment and nowadays we are working in $70m^2$ (four rooms) with two under water treadmills and every modality we dreamed of thirteen years ago!

The clinic

The clinic sees about 10 – 15 cases per day (50 – 75 per week), employing two full-time and one part-time veterinarians. We regularly have Masters or Doctoral students with us as well. The caseload consists of 30% post-surgical orthopaedics, 50% geriatric and/or osteoarthritis, 10% neurologic post-surgery cases, and 10% diverse problems.

Most of our cases are referred from within Vetmeduni (70%) and the rest from private practice. Usually the patients are referred with a full diagnosis of the underlying disease. If not, we make the diagnosis before the physiotherapy commences. The first visit includes a full clinical, neuro, ortho and physiotherapy examination. Based on the findings, the treatment plan will be developed. Most dogs come for therapy twice a week. Before each treatment session, an evaluation of the actual state of the animal is made and we decide if the treatment plan fits or has to change for that day.

We have fixed prices: One for the first examination (more expensive), and then a fixed price for each physical therapy session thereafter.

Barbara's strengths

I think that one of the important reasons as to why I have been successful was that I was very persistent during the first years. When I started, most veterinarians were of the opinion that physiotherapy is only needed if the surgery has failed. So I spent a lot of time explaining the benefits that physio can offer. One further point is the close cooperation between the vets at our clinics and the physiotherapists.

Maintaining and upgrading skills

We are doing a lot of research ourselves and we learn a lot from the research of other working groups as well. The contact between other physiotherapists and us is also very important. Naturally, we read articles and books that are published on the topic, and attend relevant congresses, such as the biannual symposium of the International Association of Veterinary Rehabilitation and Physical Therapy (IAVRPT) and the annual Veterinary European Physical Therapy and Rehabilitation Association (VEPRA) meeting. Moving forwards, I will continue with my research work, focusing on the biomechanics of rehabilitation.

Education

I think that much improvement is needed in regards to education. There are excellent course like the CCRP [certified canine rehab practitioner course available through the University of Tennessee in the USA and in Europe], which provide excellent education for beginners. However, I would like to see a more advanced course offered here in Europe.

The future of animal rehab

In the future, I would be happy to see created a European Diplomate College for Sports Medicine and Rehabilitation like in the USA. I hope to see more and more specialist vets, nurses, and technicians working together. More research is needed to prove and develop our treatment modalities.

Thoughts on why some practitioners or facilities fail

In my opinion one of the biggest problems is that persons with insufficient education try to perform physiotherapy. I often hear that physiotherapy is started without a correct diagnosis of underlying problems or is only done by non-veterinarians without the supervision of a vet. I think that close cooperation between vets and physiotherapists is necessary for successful practice. This is a statement of principal only, and is only true in countries that allow non-veterinarians to work as animal physiotherapists. In many European countries, only vets are allowed to perform animal physiotherapy.

Words of advice
Be serious in your practice. Make a solid diagnosis. Develop adequate treatment plans. Be critical regarding the success of your treatments. Never stop learning.

Beth Williams,

PT, GCS (geriatric clinical specialist),
APT (animal physical therapist)
K9 Wellness Center
Reno, Nevada, USA
www.k9wellnesscenter.com
Phone: (775)750-5087
E-mail: k9rehab@aol.com

In the beginning...

I began treating animals by working with my own Rottweiler puppy, "Nitro," during his recovery from surgery for severe hip dysplasia. In 1998 he had an experimental procedure (bilateral d'arthroplasty) using a bone graft from the iliac crest to reshape the hip joint, since he was not a good candidate for the more traditional surgical approaches. As a therapist, I knew that the instructions for crate rest (i.e. "bed rest" in human therapy) were important for healing, but that rest alone would not return him to optimal function. So, I did keep him from running/playing, but I also walked him in the yard with a sling to support his rear end, applied cold packs to his hips, did some massage and gentle range of motion exercises, and closely observed his progress.

Initially, the veterinarian thought I was a nut who was obsessed with her dog, as I would report details such as "he now sits with his hocks eight inches apart," and "only holds his left leg up every five to six steps." I explained that as a therapist I am trained to observe, note, and record movement and changes in function, and I admitted that I was not strictly following his crate-rest-only instructions.

Nitro's surgeon was impressed with his recovery and put me in contact with the owner of a local dog daycare who wanted to provide rehabilitation services at her facility. Working with my own dog is one thing, but working with someone else's pet is another, and I knew that I needed some more formal education. Before accepting any client referrals, I attended the first class for physical therapists and veterinarians on animal physical therapy and rehabilitation at the University of Tennessee in 1999. And so, K9 Wellness Center was born!

And now?

I'm still at K9 Wellness Center, a freestanding outpatient clinic. I see a mixed caseload of approximately 30 patients a week: 30% ortho, 30% neuro, 25% geriatric, and 15% fitness/conditioning/weight loss. I do occasionally treat felines and equines, despite the business name! It's just me. I have no assistants, or aides, or other staff members at this time.

Practice details...

Patients are referred for physical therapy services by their veterinarian. State statutes require a written prescription for therapy. If someone "finds" me through the Internet or by word of mouth, they can print a referral form from my website, or I will fax a referral form and note to their DVM. Once we have a referral and medical records, we start with an initial appointment to evaluate the dog's mobility, strength, range of motion, healing from surgery, pain levels, activity tolerance, etc. and establish therapy goals based on the dog's age, breed, medical status, "occupation" and owner's expectations. Sometimes the goal is just for the dog to walk outside in the yard for voiding, sometimes the goal is for the dog to return to hunting or competition in agility, and sometimes the goal is for the dog to return to "work" as a police dog, search and rescue, or service dog.

Patients generally start with visits once or twice a week, and gradually decrease to once every two to four weeks, depending on the dog's status, owner's ability to comply with a home program, transportation, finances, etc. Occasionally, I do home visits or visits at the veterinarian's clinic if the animal cannot be safely transported or is too stressed when out of his/her environment (this is especially true for cats).

Dogs that have had an uncomplicated orthopedic surgery may require 4-10 therapy visits over a 1-3 month period to return to function. Complicated cases (such as multiple fractures or back surgery) may require therapy for 4-6 months. Dogs with progressive neurological problems and geriatric dogs with advanced arthritis may attend therapy intermittently for the rest of their lives, with goals of maintaining optimal mobility and quality of life. As these dogs decline, I often help owners obtain and fit adaptive equipment such as slings, wheelchairs, protective boots or braces, incontinence supplies, etc. And I sometimes serve in helping owners evaluate their pet's quality of life and support them as they make end of life decisions.

Because I work alone, I only have one client in the clinic at a time. Visits generally last 45-60 minutes and typically include some physical modality (heat/cold, electrical stimulation, ultrasound, and/or low-level laser), manual therapy/massage, therapeutic exercises for balance, strength, flexibility, endurance, and instruction of the owner in a home program. I have a 4' deep indoor pool for swimming, and a flat-bottomed hot tub for standing/walking in warm water and "jet massage." I frequently use a land treadmill, and teach owners how to safely exercise their dogs at home using a treadmill to control speed, distance, incline, distractions, etc.

An individualized exercise program might include stepping over or going under obstacles, balancing on unstable surfaces (balance boards, air cushions, therapy balls), moving forward/backward/sideways/circling at various paces, walking up/down ramps or climbing stairs. And I provide and frequently update a written exercise program that the owner can safely perform at home with a minimum of equipment.

For healthy dogs, no referral is necessary to participate in exercise or fitness training, so they schedule an initial visit and typically attend one to two visits a week. Fitness training may include swimming, land treadmill training, coordination training using balance boards, balls, etc. "Danny," a golden retriever, has been swimming at K9 Wellness every one to two weeks since he was two, and he just turned ten!

Initially, his owner found that swimming was a great way to burn off his "puppy energy." As he matured, swimming the day before a rally-o competition helped him maintain focus and helped him win his championship. And now he swims as a low impact way to exercise his aging joints and maintain cardiovascular fitness.

Basically, I bill per visit. The initial evaluation is one charge and ongoing visits are another, regardless of time or modalities used. If clients have pet insurance or are involved in a lawsuit, they pay me at the time of service and I provide an invoice for their claim. I do give a significant discount on services to rescued animals in foster care and/or shelters, anywhere from 50% - 100%, depending on the circumstances.

Background skills and keeping up-to-date

I am a board certified specialist in geriatric physical therapy, and I find that having worked with elderly humans is good preparation for working with elderly dogs. They tend to have the same issues—decreased strength, mobility, flexibility and endurance, and similar diagnoses (arthritis, hip replacements, disc disease, etc.) Instructing the caregivers of both elderly humans and animals in a home program and appropriate daily activities is integral to their care. Having worked with patients who have impaired communication abilities (very young and developmentally delayed pediatric clients and adults who have had a stroke or brain injury) has taught me to be very observant and to communicate non-verbally. Manual therapy is key to successful physical therapy, and continuing education classes in (human) myofascial release, acupressure, joint mobilization and Aston-Patterning have greatly improved my palpation and treatment skills for animals.

I have a M.A. degree in counseling and educational psychology, and I have been well trained in compassionate listening skills. I am also a licensed prayer practitioner through the Centers for Spiritual Living and find that having my own strong spiritual base allows me to be a calm and healing presence in stressful situations.

Early on, I attended the initial course in Tennessee, followed by classes in Canada, as there was not much offered in the U.S. To keep up to date, I attend the annual Wild West Veterinary Conference yearly and focus on the orthopedic, neurological and behavioral lectures. I have attended three International Symposiums on Rehabilitation and Physical Therapy in Veterinary Medicine over the years. I am always on the lookout for advanced courses, such as the Symposium on Therapeutic Advances in Animal Rehabilitation scheduled for June 2013.

I read about animal behavior and learning in books and online, and I subscribe to the Whole Dog Journal. I take lots of positive reinforcement training classes with my own dogs and show up as a spectator at different types of competition (obedience, agility, fly-ball, luring, Rally-O, dock diving, etc) to appreciate the physical requirements of different sports.

Referrals and advertising

About 75% of the referrals I receive are from primary care veterinarians. The orthopedic specialty clinic in the area now has their own therapy services provided by veterinary technicians, but they do still occasionally refer neurological or complicated orthopedic cases. The other 25% find me through word of mouth, website, marketing booths at events, etc. and then we obtain a referral from the DVM.

I advertise in the yellow pages and have a website that "Googles" well if someone is searching for animal physical therapy in the area. My website is also "linked" with other websites—local trainers and rescue groups and with national companies that provide specialty services to disabled pets (i.e. HandicappedPets.com and AblePet.com). I have advertised in local newspapers and animal magazines with minimal success. I get exposure to the general public through booths at pet friendly community events, which do not generally yield immediate results but do generate "name recognition." And I have gained clients through classes that I co-teach and market with a dog trainer friend (i.e. exercises for you and your dog, how to massage your dog, treadmill training, etc.).

Referrals from satisfied clients to their friends/family are an invaluable marketing tool that takes time to build. Creating strong relationships with today's clients can result in future patients when they obtain their next pet.

Strengths that have made K9 Wellness Center successful
I didn't quit my day job immediately! I started very part time (lunch hours, after work, on Saturday mornings, etc.) with a partner who owned a dog day care and boarding facility, so I had very little overhead for the first four years. Initially, I did not take a salary, and we used the profits to purchase "pre-owned" equipment, including a hot tub, above ground pool, ultrasound and laser. For a while, I treated animals in a motor home parked in front of the daycare to provide a quieter/calmer treatment environment while still having access to the hydrotherapy and exercise areas indoors. I also collaborated with another animal physical therapist in the area and provided services through her business at a veterinary specialty clinic, which did generate some income. My partner and I eventually parted ways, and I moved into a 1200 square foot space in an industrial complex, where I still practice today.

I am fortunate to have a very supportive and "handy" husband who has built ramps, balance boards, treatment tables, and who installs and maintains equipment for me. I work a lot of hours—probably 50-60 hours per week doing the laundry, cleaning, bookkeeping, filing—in addition to seeing clients and updating their medical records. Low overhead and having no employees allows me to keep my prices low enough that people are able to afford my services even in a slow economy. That's the financial stuff....

On a professional level, I have created strong relationships in the animal care community—with veterinarians and their staff, local animal rescue groups and shelters, positive reinforcement dog trainers, pet food/boutique owners, groomers, etc. I am very respectful of the veterinary professionals I work with, and clearly communicate that I feel fortunate to have the opportunity to "play on their field" and use my skills to assist their clients/patients.

On a personal level, my clients know that I really do care about them and their pet's well-being. I am willing to come early or stay late to see them, to loan them equipment if needed or help them order something, to make financial considerations/arrangements, etc. I listen to their stories, appreciate the bonds they have with their pets, and become part of their support network to help them through their pet's illness or injury.

Greatest struggle

My greatest struggle is in educating the veterinary professionals and the public that animal physical therapy is available in our area, that I am a "real therapist," and that physical therapy facilitates optimal recovery from surgery/injury in animals as well as humans. I often use the analogy that a human would not have a joint surgery, be placed on bed-rest for six weeks, and then released to play tennis with no conditioning or rehabilitation.

Why do other facilities / practitioners fail?

They may start with too much overhead and are not profitable soon enough to keep going. If done in a veterinary practice, there may be an unrealistic expectation of higher charges and billing rates. This is a very labor-intensive business and you can only effectively treat so many clients in so many hours. Therapists may be doing this as a "second job" around their full time (human) therapy job, which can overwhelm and lead to burn out. Lastly, to generate a full-time caseload in this area requires a broad referral base, and it takes a lot of time and effort to create strong relationships with many primary care clinics.

Advice

If you are just getting started, team up with an experienced practitioner and benefit from their mistakes and learning curve! Take classes (in person and online) in animal anatomy, movement, common diagnoses, etc. Spend time in veterinary clinics, shelters, and training venues. Educate yourself on animal learning, behavior and training as well as the physical aspects of veterinary care. Be realistic about your budget, and don't saddle yourself with a lot of payments for equipment that won't generate a comparable amount of revenue. As a therapist, my most valuable assets are my medical knowledge, my "hands-on" skills, and my ability to observe/evaluate movement. I then use that information in creating individualized effective exercise programs which do not require having a lot of expensive equipment.

If you want to grow your business, find a niche and be prepared to donate some of your time to attract new clients. Give a free class on conditioning and exercise for an agility club, provide pro bono or discounted therapy for animals at the local shelter, have a booth at animal friendly community events. Offer to write an article for local publications on "safe exercise in hot/cold weather," or "how therapy for geriatric animals helps keep them moving well." If you work out of a veterinary clinic, create relationships with veterinarians in the area so they are comfortable referring their clients/patients to you for therapy services without fearing that they will lose their clients completely.

Reflections

It has been very interesting to watch the development of this profession. When I started in 1999, there was no legal definition of animal physical therapy in Nevada. Upon consulting the state board of physical therapy examiners, the attorney general ruled that "physical therapy" applied only to human clients. So I called what I did "animal rehabilitation," and coordinated my care closely with referring veterinarians to avoid any implication that I was practicing veterinary medicine. The Nevada State Board of Veterinary Medical Examiners had previously created a working relationship with chiropractors that also treated animals. In 1994 the board graciously asked me and another physical therapist to participate as they drafted legislation that created an "animal physical therapist" license under their jurisdiction. It is always interesting to talk to professionals from other states (and countries) about the different rules and regulations around providing physical therapy to animals.

National news programs about "new" laser treatment for animals and veteran military dogs needing special care result in many phone calls from people eager to help their pets enjoy a long, happy life. Pictures of dogs in "wheelchairs" on social media sites continue to increase public awareness of how therapy services can benefit our animal friends. As companion animals have moved off the ranch/farm and into our homes, they have become part of our families and moved into our hearts. My clients are dedicated to the health and well-being of their pets, and so am I.

Thanks for giving me the opportunity and impetus to sit down and reflect on "what a long strange trip it's been." In looking back, I see how I have been prepared for this unique work through many personal and professional experiences and connections. I am so blessed to do what I love for a living!

Brian John Sharp,

MSc (VetPhys), BSc (Phys), BSc (Biol),
PGCertEd, PGDipHealthEd, MCSP, HPC Reg, ACPAT (A)
Canine Physio
www.caninephysio.co.uk
Uxbridge, Middlesex, England
Phone: 07960 091698
Email: caninephysio@yahoo.co.uk

Brian's credentials

- Queen Mother Hospital for Animals (Royal Veterinary College)—Small animal hospital, part-time consultancy role working with vets/nurses on wards, reviewing and advising on hydrotherapy referrals, outpatient clinics reviewing and monitoring discharged animals and treating referred animals from local vet practices.

- Canine Physio (private practice)—Working to referrals from local vet practices (small animals only). Offering assessment, physiotherapy treatment, rehabilitation, hydrotherapy. Associated with two local hydrotherapy pools—at one I have dedicated pool time to carry out hydrotherapy/aquatic physiotherapy on my own patients; at the other I have an outpatient clinic.

- Dogs Trust (Harefield)—Voluntary work advising and performing treatments on any rescued dogs requiring physiotherapy/rehabilitation.

- Teacher/lecturer on various courses about small animal physiotherapy. Course leader for the UK based Veterinary

Nurse Rehabilitation Therapist course (a course I developed myself).

- Author of several chapters and journal articles on the subject of small animal physiotherapy

Brian's journey

As a child I had always wanted to be a vet and was very dismissive of other career options. I had always loved animals, and the only reading I ever did was always about them (fact or fiction). My mum has many drawings I did as a very young child, generally of animals, but I also remember doing drawings of skeletons at quite a young age, trying to learn the names of the bones.

However, when I was studying for my final exams at school (age 17-18), my dad became terminally ill, and I ended up applying for medical school instead of veterinary school. Because of his illness and the upset and distraction caused by it, my exam results were not good enough to get me into medical school, so I did a biological science (zoology and physiology) degree instead, with the aim of applying for veterinary school after.

In those days (mid 1970s) very few mature students were accepted onto first degrees, so I was unsuccessful with my subsequent veterinary application, and my career took a very different path. I started working in medical microbiology (three years), then took a postgraduate teaching qualification and subsequently worked in health education for nine years. During this time my wife and I became involved in dog showing, and I studied for a dog breeding certificate, learning a lot about conformation, anatomy, genetics as well as the essentials of breeding dogs. Needless to say, we never actually bred a litter, but we had a small amount of success in the show ring with our Golden Retrievers.

My final job in health education developed into more of a management role and in spending all my working time writing reports and attending committee meetings, which eventually persuaded me to consider retraining. Having an interest in anatomy, sports and with my background in physiology, a career in physiotherapy seemed to be the perfect path for me (I had no idea animal physiotherapists even existed then). Fortunately, my wife was fully supportive of my desire to change careers even though at 35 years of age it meant leaving a well-paid job to receiving a small bursary accompanied by long hours of study.

In those days (late 1980s) most physiotherapy training schools in the UK were attached to hospitals (not universities) and most only accepted female school-leavers. Being a "very mature man," I didn't readily fit the bill, but fortunately, my local training school had a very different attitude and welcomed both men and mature students, and I managed to get accepted onto the next available course.

I have to say I loved my physiotherapy training and won the year prize twice out of the three years. I think the realization that I had to succeed because this was really the last throw of the dice for me as far as a change of career was concerned, caused me to work incredibly hard. After qualification, I worked for a variety of local hospitals, gradually becoming more senior and obviously attending a huge number of CPD courses. Even though I had always wanted to be a vet, I had never really considered using my physiotherapy training to treat animals, and I didn't even realize that was a possibility until years later.

Brian's awareness

I gradually became aware that some physiotherapists worked with animals, but on looking into it a bit more, the training seemed pretty poor at that time; there was no real structure to it, and frankly, it seemed a bit elitist with "qualified" animal physiotherapists often not very helpful, and they seemed to primarily work with horses (whereas my main interest was, and always has been, with small animals). In 2000, the Royal Veterinary College (RVC) started the MSc in Veterinary Physiotherapy, and at last there was a formal recognized training. I applied for the first intake. The first course filled up very quickly, largely with physios already working with animals, so I did not get a place on that first course, but was successful for the second intake in 2001.

I thoroughly enjoyed my training and even enjoyed working with horses, although not being a "horsey" person, I struggled with a lot of the jargon associated with keeping and riding horses, so I felt a little out of my depth when dealing with owners. There were very few veterinary physios specializing in canine/feline physio at that time, but I decided early on this was the area I wanted to specialize in myself, and I felt much more comfortable in the presence of dogs and their owners.

The continuing work

While doing my MSc I continued to work in my local hospital physiotherapy department, working primarily in musculoskeletal outpatients and pain management, although during the eight years or so I had previously worked in hospitals, I worked in just about every physiotherapy specialty at some stage (most at a senior level), and all this experience has been invaluable in my animal work. Once I had completed my veterinary physio training in 2004, I continued to work in human physio while I started to build up my private practice in veterinary physio. This was incredibly slow to build as, at that time, most small animal vets had little experience working with physios, so I had to gradually gain their confidence while establishing a client list.

In 2005 I applied to the RVC to do a PhD related to cruciate disease, stifle biomechanics and rehabilitation. At the same time I started working part-time at the small animal hospital (QMHA) at the RVC, working on the wards and advising the vets and vet nurses about physiotherapy and rehabilitation, and I really enjoyed this aspect of my work.

Unfortunately, the main emphasis of the PhD study was the design of a technique using fluoroscopy to monitor stifle biomechanics. My background had not prepared me very well for this type of study (it was really more of an engineering study), and I received very little help from my supervisors as it was not their specialty either. I stuck at it for 18 months but then made the decision to give it up. Because it was going to involve such a huge time commitment to complete the PhD, it became a simple choice really between giving up all my clinical work (privately and at the small animal hospital) and achieving the PhD (and probably going into academia), versus giving up the PhD and concentrating on my clinical work. Because I had spent a huge amount of money and time training to become a veterinary physiotherapist, I wanted to concentrate on the clinical work, and fortunately, the decision was a good one as my private practice has grown well, and I have continued to work at the small animal hospital helping to develop the physio/rehab role there. I have also become very involved in teaching and lecturing about veterinary physio and rehab and have since developed a modular course to equip vet nurses to be more effective in their rehabilitation role.

The full circle

Strangely, I feel my career has gone full circle from the time when I was ten years old and wanted to be a vet. Although I'm still not a vet (and never will be now), I actually think I have a better job, helping animals get better without the horrible aspects of being a vet. I am also using all my previous training in physiology, zoology and teaching. Even my previous jobs in microbiology and health education have proved useful on occasions. I do enjoy my work; there's nothing better than spending time cuddling up to a dog (sorry, I mean treating a dog) and knowing you are improving its quality of life (as well as that of its owners).

Brian's work today

At the QMHA I work on the wards and also have a consultation/treatment room from where I run my outpatient clinics. I am the only physiotherapist there (working two days per week), but I work with, and advise a team of specialist neuro/rehab vet nurses, orthopaedic nurses and specialist vets.

In my private practice I work alone (although I often have student physios, vet nurses and others spending time with me to observe my work). I generally treat animals in their own home, occasionally in vet practices or at hydrotherapy pools. Each week I see approximately 8-10 home patients, 12 hydrotherapy patients and 6-12 patients at the QMHA (ward and outpatients), although this can be quite variable. At a rough guess, over the course of a week, I would say my caseload breakdown would be 35% Ortho, Neuro 25%, Geriatric/arthritic 35% and the remaining "other" 5%.

The payoff

I have trouble with the pricing of my treatments because basically I'm a lousy businessman and charge much less than many of my counterparts do. Because I enjoy the work and want to really help the animals/owners in my care, I do whatever I can for them and only charge the bare minimum.

- I have a flat rate charge for initial assessment visits and another for on-going treatments.

- I make no additional charges for travel unless the distance/time involved is substantial.

- I loan equipment at no charge, and the only additional charges I make are for any "usable" items (such as electrodes, gel, splinting materials).

- At the hydrotherapy pool I charge the same for a session as a home visit. I then have to pay the pool from that income (so that my actual income per patient is quite small).

- At the Dogs Trust I make no charge whatsoever for any interventions. This is the same for other rescue dogs I treat.

- At the QMHA the charge is made by the hospital and there is an "initial assessment" charge, and "subsequent treatment" charge. The QMHA then pays me at an hourly rate.

- At the QMHA I also do quick hydrotherapy checks prior to dogs starting their hydrotherapy programme (this is to ensure the referral is appropriate and for me to assess whether any further physiotherapy intervention might be appropriate). There is no charge made by the hospital for this service.

Working the business

In my private practice I receive referrals from local vet practices that know me and respect the work I do. I occasionally receive referrals from new practices that rapidly become part of my network. I also receive emails/calls from owners who have heard about me (word of mouth) and want me to assess/treat their animal, but in these cases I have to make contact with their vet to get permission to treat (which is generally no problem) so those vet practices also get to know about me as well.

Once I have performed my initial assessment, I discuss my findings with the owner (and occasionally the vet) to explain what intervention I believe is required, the timescale for treatment, etc. I then start treatment and continue to visit as required until the owner and I are happy with the outcome. This may involve a couple of treatment sessions (maybe working on a rehabilitation schedule) or on-going treatments at intervals (maybe once, twice or three times a week for acute injuries, or once every two or three weeks for chronic conditions). I treat a lot of elderly dogs with arthritic conditions and may treat them on a regular basis for months or years to maintain their mobility, and I've had a great deal of success over the years treating this particular group of patients.

When I first started in private practice the vast majority of contacts was from owners themselves who had found out about me, and I began treatment after gaining the appropriate approval from their vet. Over the years, this has changed, as an increasing number of vets have got to know about me, and today most of my clients are referred by vets (local first opinion practices as well as referral practices), although I still get contacted directly by owners on occasions. I also receive referrals from the hydrotherapy pools I work with, although this still necessitates contacting the animal's vet for permission for me to treat.

At the QMHA I receive most of my referrals from the specialists who also work there (mainly orthopaedic and neurological), who refer to me following initial consultation or surgery. I have also developed a "following" of local vets who refer their patients to me at the hospital (in the same way they would refer to one of the specialist vets for an orthopaedic opinion, for instance).

Brian's marketing strategy

I have a website (one of the first vet physios in the UK to have one) and whereas this was very effective in gaining work initially, most of my colleagues now have one as well, so it is certainly less effective these days. I have advertising leaflets which I have available at hydrotherapy pools, local vet practices, etc. In the past I have also attended events at dog charities, etc. Today, I actually do very little direct advertising as I get sufficient work from my friendly vet practices.

I am also advertised via the website of my professional organization (ACPAT). As with my own website, this was very useful initially when there were low numbers of members, but these days there are many members, and as the advertising is done on an alphabetical basis, being an 'S' means I am several pages down the list (and frankly, who is going to bother looking down several pages of names to select someone who seemingly has the same qualifications, etc. as everyone else?). Hence, I virtually get no contact these days from this source.

At the QMHA, advertising is done via the hospital. I have direct input into the advertising literature and website content.

Basically, I believe the best advertising by far is doing a good job and getting patients better. When owners and vets see first-hand the improvement in their pets, they are much more likely to refer again. Even in the cases that do not necessarily get better, if the owner/vet sees that you are:

- Doing your very best
- Explaining your reasoning behind your interventions
- Trying to involve them in the treatment programme as much as possible
- Being cooperative with treatment schedules/times, etc.
- Providing a good service at a reasonable price...

The clients will come back and also recommend you to other owners (and vets will continue to refer).

Brian's thoughts on why some fail
There is still a lack of acceptance from some vets regarding the benefits of physiotherapy and fear on the part of some vets of losing control over their clients. Plus, I feel there are now too many people "qualifying" as vet physios; in the UK there are far too many "training courses" for veterinary physios.

When I started in veterinary physio, ACPAT was the only organization involved in this aspect of veterinary care, so even though many vets may not have been aware of physio, it was relatively easy for them to access a properly qualified veterinary physiotherapist if they wanted one. Since then there have been a multitude of courses set up qualifying people (from various backgrounds) as rehabilitation therapists (most of these courses have come over from the USA), and hydrotherapy training has also developed. Personally, I don't have a problem with these courses, as they do not purport to "qualify" people as veterinary physiotherapists, so there is a distinction between the "physiotherapist" title and the "rehabilitation therapist" or "hydro therapist" title, allowing easy distinction by the owner or vet.

However, in recent years certain organizations in the UK have run courses to actually "qualify" people as veterinary physiotherapists (without them already being a qualified human physio with all the knowledge and skills that comes with it), and it has now reached a point where there are several of these courses running, together with a multitude of "professional" organizations that have developed from them, each purporting to be "the" organization for veterinary physiotherapists, yet most of whom only have a handful of members. This has led to:

- Massive resentment among properly qualified veterinary physiotherapists, especially ACPAT members who are by far the majority and the only ones who are actually qualified human physiotherapists having to work to recognized standards and maintain CPD requirements, etc.

- Confusion, as we see the status and the title of the properly qualified physiotherapist being effectively stolen by these other groups/courses. As a result, owners are employing vet physios, believing them to be of the same standard and training as those who treat them in hospital, only to be employing someone who has a great deal less training and experience.

- Financially, these other "vet physios" can also charge less for their services, as they do not have the same overheads in membership/registration costs, insurance, CPD requirements, etc. as ACPAT members.

Frankly, I fear for the future of veterinary physiotherapy in the UK unless the veterinary profession starts to fully respect and acknowledge the skill set of the properly qualified vet physio. Unfortunately, most of these "other courses" have been set up and organized by vets themselves, who have no or little training in physiotherapy or rehabilitation. So realistically, as things stand at present I can see no light at the end of the tunnel, apart from a steady "dumbing down" of the veterinary physiotherapist role.

Brian's honesty and strengths

I think there are several reasons why clients/vet practices continue to use my services:

- I always try to do my best for the patient and the owner. I am always honest with the owner and explain fully what I believe I can do for their pet. If I don't believe I can help much then I will tell them that.

- I keep my prices reasonable (probably much cheaper than most of my colleagues) because ultimately, I am doing this work to help the animals in my care, and earning money (although important) comes second to me. I do not charge for loaning equipment or completing insurance forms. I believe this approach is appreciated by owners, but not particularly by my wife or my bank manager!

- I always try to be as flexible as possible in arranging appointments. I will often see patients in the evenings and also have a regular hydrotherapy slot every Sunday when I treat many of my clients in the water. I make no additional charge for working "out of hours," and I do think owners are appreciative of the personal input I provide.

- I have become involved in doing a lot of teaching to vets and vet nurses and have always promoted my professional organization (ACPAT) as the primary organization that vets should work with. I continue to receive emails from vets and nurses who have attended my courses in the past, asking my advice about further training or specific cases they are struggling with, and I always try to help as much as possible.

- I have a vast amount of skills originating from my time working as a human physiotherapist. I have attended many courses and worked in many different areas of physiotherapy, and all this experience and knowledge has been invaluable in my animal work.

- I am also qualified as a teacher, having completed a postgraduate teaching qualification and working in health education many years ago. The skills and knowledge I learned from these experiences have prepared me very well for my teaching role in animal physiotherapy.

- I have also completed several courses in animal acupressure, which I have used occasionally in my clinical work.

Some of the challenges Brian faced

When I first started in private practice it took several years to build up a name and reputation, and so it was necessary to continue working as a human physio most of the time to ensure some income. Although this was only about nine years ago, getting vets interested in physiotherapy was difficult, as most knew little about it, and I believe many regarded physiotherapy as an alternative to their work, rather than a complimentary service to help their work. Fortunately, I do believe this is changing. As my reputation grew, more practices wanted to work with me, and gradually "'word-of-mouth" from owner to owner and vet to vet started getting me more cases as well.

I think my biggest disappointment in this work was when I discovered that a "fellow" ACPAT member had suddenly taken over the physiotherapy provision of a large practice that I had been involved with for years, and also a patient I was actively treating at the time. This was despite being aware of my involvement. Unfortunately, this happens, but it drummed home to me that clearly some people care more about making money than what is morally right and respecting their fellow professionals. I like to think I would never do anything similar to a colleague.

In addition, the UK learning opportunities for veterinary physiotherapists as a whole are quite poor. ACPAT has an annual seminar covering canine and equine work, but most other courses organized for members are strongly slanted to equine work.

International conferences are generally organized in the USA, which, because of the costs involved, makes it very difficult for UK physios to attend. Fortunately, there are plenty of human physiotherapy courses available throughout the UK that are obviously open for ACPAT members to attend; it is then the responsibility of the individual vet physio to determine how to adapt this information to their animal patients.

Brian's advice for newcomers

Have respect for others you work with, whether that is other vet physios, vets, vet nurses, or owners. Treat them the way you would wish to be treated, and acknowledge that they have their own unique skills that can be used effectively in cooperation with your own.

Treat your patients the way you would wish your pet to be treated and you will quickly gain the respect of their owners. Be flexible, understanding and cooperative with owners, as they may be struggling to cope with the demands of their injured or disabled pet.

Take time to learn about the animals you are planning to treat, their behaviour as well as their pathologies; remember, they can bite, kick and scratch if they are fearful of you. Become comfortable and confident around animals and learn how to handle them in a calm, assured way. Performing physiotherapy with animals often requires them to feel relaxed in your presence.

Keep up to date with developments in veterinary medicine/surgery as well as physiotherapy, but remember having vast amounts of knowledge/skills must be combined with the performing of actual clinical work. You can learn a huge amount by doing assessments and treating animals, seeing what works and what doesn't. Be flexible and adaptable in the way you carry out your treatments, and this will help you learn.

Acquire as much clinical experience as possible treating humans before embarking on a veterinary physio career. Too many newly qualified human physiotherapists are moving straight into animal work without developing a solid grounding in the principles and practice of physiotherapy with people. Human patients can provide you with lots of useful feedback about your treatment techniques that animals cannot. Although the treatment of animals often demands a different approach than treating humans, if you can get it right with people, you're much more likely to succeed with your animal patients.

The future of animal physiotherapy?

Unfortunately, I am not hopeful that the future is bright for animal physiotherapy in the UK unless things start to change soon. In the UK, the situation regarding qualifications for animal/veterinary physiotherapists is very confusing, and there are no legal requirements for someone to work as one—as long as the vet is happy with you, no actual qualifications are required. However, this must be countered by the fact that the veterinary profession as a whole is becoming much more aware of the benefits of physiotherapy and rehabilitation; the fact that it is becoming commonplace to find some elements of physiotherapy included in many "pure" veterinary courses/conferences; that physiotherapists are increasingly being employed directly by veterinary practices/referral/rehab centres or being utilized via referral.

But although physiotherapy is becoming more accepted within veterinary practice, unfortunately, it is likely to remain under the control of the veterinary profession, not only from the point of controlling who can treat their patients but also taking increasing control over the training of veterinary physios. This latter fact is the most dangerous, because it means non-physio professionals (vets) are training the physios of the future in a subject they are not qualified in themselves.

Brian's final thoughts

I think the only thing I would have done differently is to get started in animal practice earlier, maybe doing the training that was available in those early days (even though it was very ad hoc) and starting my practice sooner. Contrary to that though is the fact that things have actually fallen very well for me, and maybe starting earlier may not have been any advantage. I'm actually very content that I have achieved what I have in such a short period of time.

Since completing this questionnaire Brian's circumstances have now changed. He has moved with his family to another part of the UK and is now semi-retired. He continues to teach and write about small animal physiotherapy and rehabilitation and maintains a small clinical workload. However, his long-term plans are to spend more time with his family and dogs and become partially self-sufficient.

Brooke Marsh,

BPhty, MAnimSt
Holistic Animal Physiotherapy
Sunshine Coast, Australia
www.holisticanimalphysio.com.au
E-Mail: brookephysio@gmail.com

How did you get involved in animal physio, Brooke?
I have always had a passion and affinity for animals. When the Masters in Animal Physiotherapy became available in Australia, I knew this was the right path for me in 2003. Working as an Animal Physiotherapist started as a passion, and I gradually developed a business model and developed a website. Once I had completed my training, I began meeting face to face with local vets to discuss the benefits of Animal Physiotherapy. To work in a developing profession, it boils down to communication and persistence!

Gradually, I weaned off from my human private practice caseload as I started working at a veterinary specialist centre. The drive was one hour each way from Brisbane daily, just to build up my animal-caseload initially. I did a lot of voluntary work in Australia (at Australia Zoo) and overseas for animal conservation work (e.g. bears in Cambodia, elephants in Thailand). This was very rewarding and a great experience. I then went on to present at conferences as part of the veterinary specialist team. Basically, it took a lot of passion and persistence to build up a caseload and awareness, which is ongoing, of course! My passion has also led me to serving as the Chair on the Australian Physiotherapy Association - Animal Physiotherapy Group (APA – APG). This is such a privilege.

How do you practice?
I work full-time out of a veterinary specialist centre and see an average of 50 dogs a week (and some cats). The caseload is 60% orthopaedic (including geriatrics), 30% neurologic, 5% fitness and conditioning, and 5% miscellaneous cases.

I have been a solo practitioner in this practice, but I would love another animal physio to join my team. I just can't find one! However, a vet-nurse has just started with me part-time, and I am training her as my Physiotherapy Assistant.
Some of the caseload is comprised of in-house referrals (50%) and the website has been a major component for obtaining out-side referrals/local vet referrals. In Queensland, we are still reli-ant on veterinary referral for provision of service. Once they are referred, I have a standardized initial consultation fee and revisit charges, but I also provide some "unassisted" treadmill sessions at a reduced cost for cases that don't need "hands-on" or to help out financially restricted clients. It is very important to feedback to referring vets after the initial consultation, which I do reli-giously via letter, phone or email.

My main advertising investment has been my website. I've done newspaper and magazines advertising before, but I found those to not be worth it financially, as the website gets a lot of traffic, particularly with the integration of my blog, Twitter, Facebook, etc. I have done some radio and TV appearances/interviews too, which builds awareness for the community about Animal Physi-otherapy.

What have been your strengths regarding your practice?
Hard work, focusing on high quality of service, and communication has been my strategy. I am fortunate I work with a vet specialist who is pro-rehab, and gradually, I have been educating him about physiotherapy over the years. I continue to be positive and realize that the profession will take time to develop. As well, I tend to work closely with the vet nurses in-house by communicating with them regularly, and I provide training sessions and continuing education for referring vets and nurses.

I did Pilates as a human physio, which is great for rehabilitation exercises and stability training. I have a passion for combining eastern and western techniques in my treatments and have continued with acupuncture training over the years. As well, a large variety of human private practice and neurologic clinical experience over the years has provided me with knowledge and skills, which I draw upon for a wide variety of canine clients.

In your opinion, why do you think that some animal physiotherapy practitioners or facilities/departments fail?
Animal Physiotherapy is such a new profession in Australia and worldwide. It will take years to develop awareness of the rehabilitation needs of our four-legged clients. The veterinary profession does not receive much training regarding the benefits of rehabilitation and so it takes time to build an understanding.

Physiotherapists are not primary practitioners here in Queensland, and that makes it very difficult to build general awareness of the service, and as a general rule, we cannot charge what we do in human clinic. We are also not allowed to diagnose, and therefore, the full scope of our skill set is underutilized in the animal field as compared to our human clinical practice. Many Masters graduates (Master of Animal Studies in Animal Physiotherapy) have gone back to human work. I am trying to get pet insurance to cover animal physiotherapy. A few insurance companies do cover it at this stage. I think this will also help a lot.

It takes a lot of passion to stay in a new profession. It will take time, perhaps decades to build. With home, family and financial stresses, many therapists need to go back to human work. Veterinary awareness of rehabilitation is very poor, and I have heard many vets/vet clinics say that they already "do physio" (but only providing passive ROM, massage, etc.), and this is an issue.

What has been your greatest struggle or challenge in practice?

Firstly, the lack of awareness in the veterinary profession about physio and rehabilitation has been the biggest hurdle. Secondly, not being primary practitioner and requiring a referral to treat has potentially slowed the advancement of animal physiotherapy. Being a new profession there are limited numbers of qualified animal physiotherapists, and therefore, limited awareness of its existence across the board. So, generally speaking, "lack of awareness of the profession" has been most challenging.

How do you maintain or upgrade your animal physiotherapy skills & knowledge?

I partake in ongoing training by attending human courses to apply to animals. I attend and present at conferences (i.e. the Australian Physiotherapy Association), take courses, and endeavour to update myself on the latest research. I find that training staff nurses and vets helps me to be up to date with my own skills, and presenting at veterinary conferences each year keeps my knowledge fresh because of the need to research the topic I am presenting. I have recently co-presented on our APA level 1 Animal Physiotherapy course for Physiotherapists, which was a great way for me to update my knowledge and skills in order to teach this subject effectively. The Animal Physiotherapy group (APA) runs regular professional development sessions in each State, which I help to organize and attend.

What is YOUR next step as an animal physiotherapy practitioner?

I am trying to obtain assistance in my clinical practice by working with a veterinary nurse in order to help with the physical load. Also, I would like to build my rehab practice by having another trained animal physiotherapist on staff, which would allow me more time to continue to build the profession through the APG, develop an educational pathway, and build my own business. I would love to have a larger facility once I have this backup, including a pool (I have an underwater treadmill currently) and to be readily accessible by the general population. I have recently been involved in writing and teaching the level 1 of the animal physiotherapy course through the Australian Physiotherapy Association and am currently Chair of APG, working to continue developing our profession.

What do you think about the learning opportunities in the field of animal physiotherapy in Australia?

We have been working for many years to reinstate the Masters qualification through various universities around Australia since it ceased in 2007. Hopefully, this will start again in 2014. Over the last few years the committee has written the Level 1 Animal Physiotherapy course, which is the start of our educational pathway through the Australian Physiotherapy Association. This is a slow process, but we are happy to have a pathway for human physiotherapists to train as animal physiotherapists in Australia again.

After the Masters qualification there is little avenue for those of us with that degree to acquire further training. Those of us qualified spend a great deal of time training those who want to get in the profession. We have tried to run "master classes" alongside of our gatherings to assist with this process. We still have a long way to go, but I am confident there are more options now for on-going development!

What advice would you give to someone new to the field of animal physiotherapy?

Be aware of the educational pathways to become an animal physiotherapist and know that it will take time and dedication. Initially, there may not be financial rewards, so I recommend having some backup with a human caseload in that time. If the physiotherapist is passionate about working with animals, it is a fantastic job. I love my work!

What would you LIKE to see for the future of animal physiotherapy?

I would like to see physiotherapists gain primary practitioner status, which will open up our career path as it did for human physios in 1978 in Australia. Prior to this, when a medical doctor's referral was required, little was known about physiotherapy. I would like to see educational pathways built that have consistent graduate numbers. We need strength in numbers in order to build awareness of the profession in both the community and veterinary profession. Lastly, I would like to see physio become part of mainstream veterinary medicine, as it is in the human model (e.g. 97% of cruciate ligament repairs in human orthopaedics have post-operative physiotherapy).

Is there anything else you would like to comment on?

Basically, I love my animal work and have no regrets going down this path. My day-to-day work is fantastic and I am very grateful that I have options—human AND animal career paths. Perhaps the biggest difference working with animals is that they don't have the same emotional issues humans do with chronic pain. They heal quickly and are survivors. So they are very satisfying to treat! I love the path that physio has taken me on, and I'm excited about the next phase—especially with further advancement of the profession, which will make it easier for those coming through now and in the future.

Cajsa Ericson,

BSc (Chartered Physiotherapist), Licensed Physiotherapist
Approved in Veterinary Medicine by The Swedish Board of
Agriculture
www.horsepower.dinstudio.se
Phone: +46708 301033
E-mail: cajsaericson@gmail.com
Stockholm/Norrtälje – Sweden

In the beginning...

I began practicing in the human physiotherapy field in 2003, doing sports medicine and some orthopedics. That same year I started my canine and equine physiotherapy practice as well. Currently, I see more horses than dogs.

After riding and competing with horses all my life, having hunting dogs in my family, and working professionally with race horses (harness racing) for almost 10 years, I started to get deeply interested in rehabilitation and training. I couldn't find the sort of education I was looking for in the animal field, so I thought that if I study and become a physiotherapist in the human field, that I could translate it into the animal field—and that's where it started! I did, of course, become interested in humans as well...

The main reason, and the real turning point for me in wanting to learn about animal rehab/physiotherapy, was when I was grooming one of Europe's best trotters over 3-4 years. I had to really work with him so that he could stay amongst the elite trotters in the world and continue racing against the best (at that time: Mack Lobell, Peace Corps, Napoletano, Friendly Face, and Express Ride). Everything about caring for this horse—feeding, travelling around the world, training, rehabilitation, fitness, you name it—made it clear to me that the horse's success wasn't only about the animal or the trainer, but it was about the entire team. And I really enjoyed being a part of that! As well, from the day that I acquired my first Labrador retriever (that hunted elk, moose, deer, and birds), I became interested in dog training. So when I received my Physiotherapy BSc, I just started practicing on animals. As a result of my contacts in the racing world over the years, many vets already knew me and were interested in my animal physiotherapy services. I contacted some small animal vets and got into their practices as well, and that's how it started and has grown throughout the years.

How Cajsa practices

In canine practice, I started to work by advising dog-owners, post-surgery, and on weight loss for their dogs, and I also rehabilitated their dogs. Now I'm practicing more and more on horses. My main canine business consists of fitness and conditioning, rehabilitation, and prevention services for the narcotic-detection-dogs working at the border and customs, and of course, some hunting dogs as well.

In horses, my main interest is preventing, conditioning, and rehabilitation. I find that the treatment of muscular pain is a large part of my job. The modalities I use are acupuncture with needles, low-level-laser therapy, laser acupuncture, therapeutic ultrasound, and kinesiotaping, in addition to different training methods that I utilize.

Since I still work on humans part-time, I see about 3 – 4 dogs a week and approximately 10 – 15 horses a week. I bill the client after each treatment.

How Cajsa advertises and gets referrals

I don't actually advertise! I have a not-very-well-updated web page, and business cards to hand out, but I tend to rely on word of mouth. I have done lectures and workshops that bring in new clients, and in the beginning, I put up some advertisements in stables (but I don't think they actually brought me any business, to tell the truth).

In some instances, I get referrals directly from veterinarians. The owner then contacts me, and I begin working with their animal. I maintain a good dialogue with the referring vet. Alternately, the owner contacts me directly; I examine their animal, and begin treatment. However, if the animal is lame or there is something else in which I need a veterinary diagnosis, I always refer the case to a vet before I start any treatment or devise a treatment plan.

Cajsa's strengths

I am fortunate to have the knowledge and experience from working with animals before I came into the physiotherapy field. I knew several vets and horse or dog people from before. I also think it is an advantage to utilize my human skills, and I work a lot with the rider on top of the horse, with coordination, strength training, balance training, etc. Just by knowing the human body that sits or stands behind, beside or over the top of the animal, I can advise on how the horse and animal team can better function and work together to get the best results.

Staying current

I try to attend as many conferences, clinics, and workshops that I can afford! There is such a limited amount of educational opportunities at an academic level in animal rehabilitation (especially in regards to horses), so I try to cooperate and communicate with colleagues as much as I possibly can. There is a need for more animal rehab education over all. I believe that animal rehabilitation has progressed to a point that we are now in need of new inputs, and new people to look up to. It's disappointing to look at different conference or seminar programs and see that the topics are almost identical. While it is fantastic to remember and acknowledge some of the original speakers in the field, I think it's time to expand our horizons. It would be useful to intersperse—with the "old pioneers"—knowledge, techniques, and methods from people who have been working in the field for a long time and who have acquired so much experience. I also think we need to do clinical research in order to showcase and to defend animal rehab practice.

My plan is to continue learning, establish more contacts with people interested in animal physiotherapy/rehab, and hopefully, be able to help more animals and owners with rehabilitation and injury prevention.

Why do some animal physiotherapy practices or facilities struggle or fail?

- Lack of an established contact network with veterinarians and people in the various animal sporting industries/groups when starting out
- Lack of experience and knowledge of working with animals (from the world 'outside of the animal-PT realm')
- Competition from 'alternative' practitioners

- Lack of understanding of the benefits of animal rehabilitation on the part of vets and owners
- Lack of energy and hope...

It can be really tough out there, especially in the beginning. I know for myself, I have struggled to defend my practice and animal physiotherapists as a group to vets that are sometimes skeptical about me/us and physiotherapy methods and knowledge. It can be frustrating to hear: "There is no evidence in what you are doing..."

Cajsa's advice to new practitioners
Do good work and get results! Get to know "important people" that can help with your learning and/or can help to get you started. Get to know and visit with individual vets and vet clinics. Ask if you can shadow them for a day. Be patient, it takes time!

Carrie Smith,

BScPT, CCRT, CAFCI, Cert. Sport Physio, Cert. Gunn IMS
Kemptville Physiotherapy: www.kemptvillephysio.com
Carleton Vet Services: 613-489-2525
carriephysio@bellnet.ca
Ottawa, Ontario, Canada

Cool stuff about Carrie

I practice about 60% of the time on humans (orthopaedics and sports physiotherapy) and 40% on animals (of which 90% is canine practice). I have affiliations with the University of Ottawa as the women's rugby head PT, am a member of the Canadian Physiotherapy Association (with membership in the Animal Rehab Division, Sports Division, Ortho Division), and Rugby Canada. *[Editor's note: Carries leaves out the fact that she is an integral member of the board of directors for the Animal Rehab Division of the Canadian Physiotherapy Association!]*

Carrie's beginnings

Well, around 1987 or so, I was practicing in a private orthopaedic clinic in Fort McMurray, Alberta. There was a vet in the same building, and one day she ran over and asked us if we would mind looking at a dog for her. A dog? Yes, a dog.

The dog had a spinal problem that she had not seen before and did not really know how to treat. The other PT and I looked at each other and said, "sure, why not?" The dog came in with the vet and the owners, and it was deviated through the thoracic and lumbar spine. I mean this dog was really deviated! If his nose and front feet were pointing at 12:00, then his tail and hind legs were pointing around 4:00. Well, this is a problem that humans get all the time, just ask Robin McKenzie! *(Editor's note: Robin McKenzie is a well-known Australian physiotherapist, primarily credited with developing unique treatment techniques for the spine and disc lesions in particular.)*

So we treated the dog just like we would treat a human with a spinal deviation—side glides, manual traction, electrical muscle stimulation, and some tail traction *(not generally a "human technique")*. The treatment worked very well and within two or three days the dog was straight again. The vet thought this was very cool. The owners thought this was very cool. I thought this was stupendous! Shortly after this episode, I saw an advertisement for a canine rehab course by a group named CHAP. *(Editor's note: The Canadian Horse and Animal Physical Therapists Association— the original name of the Animal Rehab Division before recognition by the Canadian Physiotherapy Association).* I decided that this was something that I needed to do...and the rest is history!

Carrie's busy canine rehab schedule

I work out of three different vet clinics—one-half day per week in two clinics and one full day per week in the third. I have the use of two rooms in each clinic. In two of the clinics, I am the only rehab practitioner. On a Saturday, I would see about fifteen dogs, and on my half days, I would see five to six. One of the vet clinics has a CCRT vet and tech, so that clinic will see more rehab patients as the other practitioners are treating them. At Cedarview Animal Hospital there is one Rehab Vet, one Rehab PT (me), and one Rehab Vet Tech. At Carleton Vet Services there is one Rehab PT (me), and one Aide. And at Osgoode Vet Services, there is just one Rehab PT (me again!). My caseload tends to break down into 60% ortho (quite a few of these would be agility dogs), 20% geriatric (mostly arthritis, stenosis, degenerative disc disease, etc.), 10% neuro, and 10% general fitness.

How Carrie practices Canine Rehab

When I started treating animals I sent around an info package to all of my local vets (including referral notes, business cards and all contact info). I send a treatment note after every treatment so the vet would know how the dog was treated. The College of Veterinarians of Ontario has pretty strict rules regarding advertising. I am not allowed to advertise to the public at all, but I can advertise directly to vets to let them know what I do and where I am. I have found the best marketing strategies to be talks to dog groups, working at agility events, and attending other dog-sports events.

In the majority of cases, veterinarians refer clients directly to me for services; however, I have had people contact me directly after rehab talks or in my human practice. One veterinary practice is a surgical practice, so every orthopaedic surgery is automatically booked for rehab. Appointments are booked through the front reception at the vet clinic, as well as all the follow-ups.

Clients generally pay a flat fee for their rehab services based on treatment time: a flat fee per 30-minute treatment and a flat fee for a 60-minute assessment. ACL surgery patients can purchase a pre-paid package (four rehab appointments, six laser treatments with tech, twelve UWT workouts, and E-stim for home use).

Carrie's strengths as a Canine Rehab Therapist

I think my biggest strength is my MANY (25+) years of human experience and multiple tools in my treatment tool kit (IMS, Acupuncture, mobilizations, exercise therapy, etc.). I get good results and most of my referrals come from word of mouth.

- I like to use Mulligan mobilizations with movement on the spine. *[Editor's note: Brian Mulligan is a New Zealand based physiotherapy that has developed unique ways to mobilize joints in conjunction with movement.]* You get the owner to do a "cookies at the hip" motion at the same time as you are doing a side glide on a spinous process, and you can get a good mobilization this way.

- I just took a visceral manipulation course for humans, and I think there are some aspects that could be used on canines. I had a cattle dog in the other day that developed a psoas problem after abdominal surgery (she ate a Kong, and they had to remove it from her small intestine). Of interest—in humans, the small intestine refers pain to the psoas muscle! So I tried a visceral treatment and she closed her eyes and drifted off to sleep while I was doing it...not sure if it helped her psoas, but I will see at her next appointment!

- IMS (intramuscular stimulation) is a huge part of my human practice, and I find it very useful with dogs as well. In humans, it is my first choice for treatment, but with dogs it is my last choice, only because it can be painful and the humans can brace themselves for it but the dogs don't "get it." The dogs I have used it on have been well known to me, and they were fine with the technique and had great results. Most of these were agility dogs with muscular injuries.

- I am certified in human acupuncture, and I find that acupuncture works well with animals. I recently purchased a laser, so I am doing a lot of laser stimulation to the acupuncture points, which I find just as effective. It takes longer than acupuncture, but I can do more points and don't lose any needles in hair!

- I work with a lot of rugby athletes, and they do a lot of proprioception and agility training. Sometimes I see what they do in practice, and then I turn it into a canine exercise!

Carrie's struggles in Canine Rehab

It is always challenging to get the vets to think about rehab as a first option for animals, as opposed to a last resort. Often I will get a referral when the vet has nothing else to offer, but if that animal had started rehab earlier they might have had a much better outcome. Often the referral comes because the owner has requested rehab, not always because it was the vet's idea to send them to rehab. The more info you can provide to the owners (like giving a talk at agility events, etc.), the more they will drive your practice. I have never had a vet deny an owner a referral, but I have had a few referrals where they really didn't think it would help the animal. It is nice to be able to send a good report back about how well the animal is doing!

My other biggest challenge is time. I am co-owner of two busy human orthopaedic private clinics, plus I work with two different rugby teams (one national team and one University team), and work in three vet practices. (I need to buy a cloning machine!) Sometimes, clients are not happy that they cannot get an appointment right away, but that's how it goes. I am not at the point where I want to be full-time working with animals, as I enjoy my human practice, and working with the national rugby team allows me to do a lot of travelling (like Rugby World Cup in New Zealand last year!). Likewise, I do not want to give up my animal practice, as that would just be insane!

How Carrie stays current and her thoughts on educational opportunities

I try to attend conferences every one to two years. As well, the Animal Rehab Division newsletter is an excellent reference for material, and I pour over that a lot! On-line sites are also good for information sharing. I love attending Therapaw's STAAR *(Symposium on Therapeutic Advances in Animal Rehabilitation; www.therapaw.com).*

When I started there were only the Canine Rehab Institute and the program at U of Tennessee available for a Certificate program in canine rehab. I took the Intro and Advanced Canine courses through the Animal Rehab Division, as well as an acupuncture point location course. Canada now has a Diploma in Canine Rehab Program for PT's, which I believe was a much-needed national program. This will help Canadian PT's to access animal rehab as a profession.

The vet/PT programs are always going to have some challenges since they are teaching to two completely diverse professions. The manual and treatment techniques that are taught are almost too simple for the PTs, and I suspect the vet information and surgical lectures are too simple for the vets, but there is really no other option. I think that advanced manual therapy courses for PTs would be a good idea, as well as things like osteopathy, bracing, and taping.

Carrie's thoughts on why some practitioners and facilities struggle in providing canine rehab and her advice for practitioners

Cost is a huge factor! I think vets over-charge for their rehab skills (i.e. their skills are not that good and they don't see big changes in outcomes as quickly as PTs do—in my opinion). I think they forget that rehab is not a one-shot deal and that the dog may have to come for several treatments. I always tell owners to book three treatments. If they have not seen a significant change by the third treatment, either I am not treating the right thing or this problem is not going to respond quickly or well to rehab (i.e. psoas problem compensating for a complete ACL tear). I feel that I should be able to make a difference in a short period of time; I know some vets who are doing many, many treatments with little success, and owners talk about poor results!

My advice:

- Get all your credentials first (Certificate or Diploma) before you start to practice.

- Vets should spend at least one day in a human practice with a PT, because human patients can give them feedback about hand pressure and joint glides when doing manual therapy.

- Don't overcharge! Look at what human clinics around your area charge for a rehab treatment. Animal rehab should not be more expensive, as the practitioners are basically "new grads."

- Spend a lot of time on assessment and re-assess at every treatment. It seems that some practitioners are doing the initial assessment, and then having the tech perform several treatments. If you don't re-assess on each visit, you will have no idea how the patient is doing. If there are no changes after the first two treatments, you are not treating the right thing, or your treatment is not effective, so don't keep doing it! The tech does not have qualifications to do your re-assessment.

- Use the "Three Treatment Rule." I tell all of my humans and owners this. If there have been no improvements after the third treatment, you are not being effective, so re-evaluate! Owners will really respect this. This does not mean that the patient is completely healed in three treatments; it just means you know you are on the right track.

I think animal rehab will continue to grow, and likely grow quickly over the next decade. Vet schools are now introducing rehab concepts and owners are becoming savvier about what is available for their animals. I think this is an exciting time to be in animal rehab! It is good to see more courses and symposiums available. I would like to see the PT schools introducing animal rehab as part of their core curriculum, and to have an animal rehab placement available for students.

One final story that Carrie wanted to share

I arrived at one of my vet clinics to find that I had a new patient scheduled—named "Sparkles." Much to my surprise, Sparkles was a two-year-old guinea pig! The owner came in with Sparkles and told me that the vet had referred him to rehab because Sparkles was not using his left hind leg. (The vet was in the clinic at the time, so I asked her about it. She said she had no idea what was wrong with the leg and had offered either an x-ray or rehab to the owner, so the owner picked rehab!).

When I assessed Sparkles, he could not walk straight and kept veering left, because the right leg was working, but not the left. On examination, there was not as much tone through the left leg and he seemed hypomobile over the lumbar spine (well, as far as I could tell anyway. My fingertip covered two to three spinal segments, so it was rather difficult to be specific!)

So, not really knowing for sure what was going on, I put my critical-thinking cap on and decided that there was probably a nerve root irritation affecting the left hind leg (he had a normal deep pain response and no incontinence). I used some very small acupuncture needles and did some points along the GV, UB and GB meridians. Sparkles home program was hanging traction, celery at the hip (side bending movements) and some jumping jacks (facilitating a landing reflex). I saw Sparkles a week later and he was walking straight! The owners were happy and so was I!

About a year later I was in the human clinic when a new patient walked in. I thought he looked familiar, and when he saw me, he said, "Hi! Remember me? I'm Sparkles' Dad!" He updated me on my favourite patient and told me that Sparkles lived out the rest of his life walking in a straight line.

Charles Evans,

MPT, CCRT
Port City Veterinary Referral Hospital, Intown Veterinary Group
215 Commerce Way, Suite 100, Portsmouth, NH 03801
www.ivghospitals.com - 603-433-0056
E-mail: cevans@ivghospitals.com

How did you start, Charlie?

I stated practicing in canine rehab in 2002, but I first became interested in the idea of physical therapy for animals in 1995 while I was working as a veterinary technician at my local veterinary hospital. I took some courses on my own (e.g. Reiki, Tellington Touch, Therapeutic Touch), but my boss was uncomfortable with applying those techniques to her practice. One of our clients, who happened to be a physical therapist, stopped in one day with a copy of *PT Magazine* that had Darryl Millis, DVM and David Levine, PT on the cover. I became more interested. I spoke to two veterinary orthopedic surgeons who thought it was a great idea and suggested I contact Dr. Bob Taylor, DVM. But they also advised that although it was a good idea (physical therapy for animals), the field of practice didn't really exist. Their advice was to get my physical therapy degree.

So I spoke to the Dean of the new PT program at Notre Dame College in Manchester, NH, who was excited about the concept of a new niche for physical therapists and a possible program that could be created to fill that niche. We gathered several teachers from both fields to collaborate; but ultimately, it was decided that there was too large a knowledge gap to make it work at the time. So I obtained my degree in physical therapy. The year after

I graduated (2001), one of the orthopedic veterinarians I had spoken to earlier asked if I would take over a part-time fledgling PT/Rehab practice he had started in order to support his post-operative patients. I did. I worked at the Dover Veterinary Hospital part time (while also practicing full-time human PT) until 2005, when I was asked to come in full time to perform PT/Rehab and support a new veterinary surgeon. This arrangement lasted until 2006, when the veterinarian that had hired me retired, and his partner decided that the space the underwater treadmill occupied would be great for an endoscopy unit! I went back to full time human PT until March of 2007, when I was hired by the Intown Veterinary Group (IVG) to work at their Massachusetts facility—the Massachusetts Veterinary Referral Hospital in Woburn, MA. This is a very large (41,000 sq. ft.) hospital, with four orthopedic surgeons and two neurologists. What an education! What an opportunity! In 2008, IVG opened its third facility in New England—New Hampshire—much closer to home for me, and I began working two days a week at Port City and two days a week at MassVet. In June of 2011, I began working at the Port City facility exclusively.

Tell us about the practice you work in now
Port City Veterinary Referral Hospital is a 24/7 emergency and referral hospital. It is a new 16,000 square foot building, with specialties in surgery, internal medicine, physical therapy and rehabilitation, radiology, cardiology, and ophthalmology. I have an underwater treadmill, cavaletti rails, balance board, physioball and rolls, rubberized flooring, pulsed magnetic field bed, low-level laser, and my hands. We also have a massage therapist who treats patients every Saturday afternoon. At Port City we employ one PT/CCRP. I have no technician. At MassVet they employ one PT/CCRP/CCRT (Amie Lamoreaux Hesbach) and one Vet/CCRT, as well as two technicians.

(Editor's note: CCRT = certified canine rehabilitation therapist; CCRP = certified canine rehabilitation practitioner. Certifications awarded by two different US canine rehab educational institutions.)

Can you tell us about the details of your practice?
We either have referrals from our in-hospital doctors or from outside referring vets. Most of the referrals come from our in-hospital doctors. We occasionally have external clients who wish to access our rehab services, and in those cases we will have one of our surgeons briefly examine the patient to be sure there are no underlying problems. Those clients are also requested to have their regular veterinarian fill out a referral form and history for our files. Once the patient is in rehab, we determine the extent of treatment and recommend some form of package and suggested duration of course of therapy.

I see 15 to 20 cases in a 16-hour workweek. The caseload breaks down to be approximately 80% orthopedic, 5% neurologic, and 15% fitness/conditioning/geriatric. Because of the inclusion of Dr. Stuart Bliss, DVM to our veterinary staff, we are now offering what we call Physical Medicine. This enables us to treat utilizing everything from massage and manual techniques to total hip replacements and everything in between!

How do you charge?
We have an individual charge for low-level laser therapy. We offer numerous packages of physical therapy and hydro-treadmill sessions, which are prepaid. We also offer individual sessions that are either prepaid or paid for immediately after the service. We have begun to break the individual sessions down by time (15-minute increments).

Do you advertise?

For the most part we depend on our website and word of mouth for advertising. We have done some outreach visits, but they are not particularly helpful. We have begun to donate a rehabilitation package (initial evaluation, six-pack of PT, six-pack of hydro) to our local public television station, and that has brought some more clients in, but not many.

Tell us more about YOU—your strengths, your struggles, and your next plans

Innovation has been a real strength of mine. I brought low-level laser therapy to Intown when I arrived in 2007. We have initiated the massage program here at Port City and will try to start a similar program at MassVet. We have also initiated the Physical Medicine program. I use a lot of manual techniques, such as strain counter strain, myofascial release and muscle energy. I also love continuing education, and I am always looking for new techniques or modalities, as I try to stay open to new options.

My biggest challenge: It has been quite difficult to promote the concept of the benefit of having rehab available and the impact that can have on a practice as a whole. Even though it doesn't bring in as many dollars as hoped all by itself, it does bring money into the practice in other realms of practice.

As for my next step and future plans, I am planning to become certified in canine acupressure. With as much manual therapy as I do, it will be an added benefit to my patients to be able to add the therapeutic modality of acupressure during a regular treatment. It's a little like Reiki; once you have been attuned, if you lay hands on a patient you will be delivering some Reiki. We have had some really good results using the manual techniques I learned from Integrative Manual Therapy that we (the facility in

Port City) are able to offer that many other rehab facilities cannot or do not.

Why do you think that some rehab facilities fail?
There are so many reasons. I have talked to many veterinary rehab practitioners who have been hired by an association of surgeons, who are completely frustrated because their own surgeons will not refer to them. There needs to be much more education of the general practitioners about the benefits of physical therapy for their animal patients—especially post-surgical and neurological. I believe that many surgeons will start a rehab practice on the side thinking that they will make a lot of money, but rehab really is not a great moneymaker! We also need to convince the surgeons that treatment doesn't stop at suture removal.

What do you think about learning opportunities in animal rehabilitation?
I have found the Therapaw workshops (Editor's note: The STAAR conference at www.therapaw.com) to be very useful. I also have found the Integrative Manual Therapy courses have been very useful, even though they are oriented toward human physical therapy. These courses are easily adaptable to dogs.

As a general comment about learning opportunities, they are slim, unfortunately. Once again the Therapaw courses have been the most useful to me. I have offered to do a course on strain counter strain for one of the Therapaw courses, but that hasn't happened yet. It would be wonderful if we were able to offer a wide variety of courses in various places, but it would take a lot of coordination and work to get it off the ground. The faculty is out there! It would be fun to see what we could do. I get many fliers from various "educational institutes," and if I were still working with humans, some very interesting courses could be taken. The same diversity of topics focused on canine or equine patients would be great to see. Courses like Laurie Edge-Hughes' *Evaluation and Diagnosis of the Cervical-Thoracic and Lumbosacral Courses*, Amie Lamoreaux Hesbach's *Neuro Rehab Course*, gait evaluation, kinesiology of gait, a whole course on the surgeries of the stifle and the follow-up rehab, and the same for the hip would be wonderful to see. Dr. Stuart Bliss, DVM just performed our (Intown Vet's) first total hip last weekend, and today he and I are going to spend an afternoon discussing the ramifications of the acetabular implant and rehab. Those kinds of things as well as manual techniques like the strain counter strain. Integrative Manual Therapy has a process of both myofascial and strain counter strain diaphragm releases that I have used on both humans and canines that get really significant results, and they are quite easy to teach to owners. These are the types of things that I would like to see brought into canine rehab education.

What do you see as the future of canine rehab?
I think the field will continue to grow rapidly. I do hope that there will be a Masters of Animal Physical Therapy offered at some point in North America. My main concern at this point is that the veterinarians are flooding the market and there are not enough PTs in the field. It's a little like being trained as a dentist and then entering the field of orthopedics by taking a short course in ortho. Physical Therapists have so much more knowledge as to how it all works, and from what I have experienced, even from the vets who do orthopedics and value physical therapy, is that they realize how little they know about rehab and are subsequently willing to just "let us do our thing."

Do you have any advice to give?

Get as much experience as possible. Stay open to new or different ways of performing therapy, and always keep adding "tools to your tool kit." I have been fortunate to have not had to consider the financial stresses of starting a practice outside of an established veterinary setting. I really like the fact that if I see something out of the ordinary or something troubling during a rehabilitation treatment that I can immediately call in a doctor for a quick consult. I would not necessarily recommend that to everyone, but for me it has made my late-blooming career much easier and less stressful.

Would you have done anything differently?

This is going to sound strange, but I would have done it just the same way. I could not have "pushed the rope" any faster than I did.

Danielle Robbins,

MS, PT, CCRT
American Dog
San Diego, CA, USA
www.AmericanDogRehab.com
AmericanDogRehab@gmail.com
Phone: 858-945-4659

How it began

In June of 2000, I began volunteering with physical therapist, Trish Penick, of Cutting Edge K9 Rehab, in San Diego, California. The focus of her practice was deep-water swimming. It charged my interest in canine rehab, and in September of 2000, I attended my first canine physical therapy course titled, "Introduction to Canine Physical Therapy." This served as the first course in what would soon be the Canine Rehabilitation Certification program through the University of Tennessee. The following year I took the second level course in the program. I spent about a year working with Trish before I started seeing canine and feline patients on a house call basis, but I continued to volunteer with Trish over the subsequent 12-months to gain more experience. In 2004, while attending an elective course on Canine Osteoarthritis in San Diego, I introduced myself to veterinarian Dr. Claire Sosna. Soon after that meeting I started to bring my own dog to Dr. Sosna for acupuncture. Within a month I began seeing one to four patients a week in her clinic, The Animal Acupuncture and Rehabilitation Center (AARC) and my practice soon grew to two and a half days per week. I went on to complete the Canine Rehab Institute's canine rehab certification program in 2006.

The practice now

I currently see patients out of AARC, an independent outpatient veterinary rehab and acupuncture facility. I am the only physical therapist on site at the one vet, four-veterinary assistant practice. At present, I see 8 – 11 patients a day and am available twice a week. Dr. Sosna sees approximately 70 – 80 patients per week. Our caseload breaks down to be about 80% orthopedic, 5% neurologic, and 15% geriatric.

Clients are billed by service. I provide manual therapy, therapeutic laser, therapeutic exercise, and home program instruction. Frequency of treatment depends on the diagnosis and/or the patient's current status and financial or scheduling constraints of the client.

Marketing

Our marketing consists of a website and placement of cards and brochures in referring vets' offices. Our referrals tend to come from specialty vets (i.e. surgeons), primary care vets, word of mouth from other clients, and those who find us via an Internet search.

Roots of success

I believe that my skill level has led to good functional outcomes and happy clients. I provide regular and timely communication with the client and referring veterinarian, and I employ comprehensive home programs.

My next steps as an animal rehab practitioner are to continue to build my knowledge regarding neurologic assessment and treatment, vestibular conditions, and advanced orthopedic assessment and treatment.

The struggles

It has been challenging to convince veterinarians of the value of early intervention after injury, and especially surgery, and of the general benefits of physical rehabilitation for a variety of different conditions that result in loss of function. It has additionally been frustrating to have to educate consumers and veterinarians about the skill and knowledge of physical therapists and how we differ from massage therapists, or others, such as lay-practitioners who claim to be qualified to provide animal rehab services. Many people (the public, veterinarians, and the lay-practitioners themselves) don't know the difference and think that anyone can provide rehab for animals! Additionally, clients with limited financial resources have prohibited some from seeking comprehensive rehab for their pets, especially in the past few years during strained economic times.

Educational opportunities

I regularly attend continuing education and participate in animal rehab chat groups. In regards to educational opportunities in the field in general, I would like more courses to be offered on the USA west coast. I'd also be interested in courses taught by physical therapists well versed in canine rehab for physical therapists only. An interest of mine would also be vestibular evaluation and treatment for the canine patient.

The future of animal rehab

I would like to see rehab to be provided only by properly trained clinicians, with indirect supervision requirements for properly trained physical therapists. I believe that there needs to be respect and recognition in the veterinary community for the skills, contributions and knowledge that the physical therapist has brought to veterinary rehabilitation.

Clear regulatory language needs to be developed that defines the scope of animal physical rehabilitation, and that eliminates "bad actors" that claim to provide "rehab" without the proper credentials to do so, or are doing so and calling it something else. Additionally, I would like to see the eradication of improper use of PT protected terms in animal rehabilitation. Consumer education is required to enlighten the public regarding what distinguishes a PT from other practitioners working in this field and why choosing a rehab team that includes a PT may enhance rehab outcomes.

I would like to see greater collaborative efforts between physical therapist and veterinarians in research, education and patient care and an animal rehab model that more closely resembles human medicine.

Additionally, I feel that a master's degree program for animal physical therapist offered in the USA would bolster the profession tremendously.

Advice
My recommendation would be to optimize one's knowledge and skills in the animal rehabilitation profession by becoming a licensed physical therapist and then attend a canine rehab certification program.

Donna LaRocque,

BScPT, CAFCI, CCRT, CERT(c)
Furry Friends Animal Rehab
Alberta & Saskatchewan, Canada
www.FurryFriendsAnimalRehab.com
Phone: 780-720-6623

How did you start?

Starting back in 2005, I began by accepting referrals from another physiotherapist with a practice three hours away and doing home visits. For a while, I worked in a stand-alone, non-vet, non-physiotherapist owned rehab practice before it closed, and then I moved on to working in a vet-owned rehab practice before it closed as well. I currently see canine patients in a general veterinary practice, trying to get the rehab piece integrated as standard protocol for all of their post-operative cases. The owner of the practice is "on board," but the others vets have not bought in yet. I continue to do home visits, and I have just recently come on board as a staff therapist at a physiotherapist-owned canine rehab facility.

Tell us about your Furry Friends animal rehab practice

I have one tech that I work with within the general vet practice, and we tend to see 10 –15 cases a week. The caseload breaks down to be 30% orthopaedics, 30% fitness, 20% geriatric, 10% neurologic, and 10% other (i.e. cancer, etc.).

I charge a flat fee for treatment. It is not based on time or modality. I do give a "free" treatment if the rehab is going to be long and I have to treat the animal quite frequently.

Clients find me mostly by word of mouth, or they are referred from an existing client. Some find me from my website. The treatment plan varies for each patient, depending on what the client is able or willing to do. Some just want a home program that is monitored; some want me to do the whole program. I can accommodate them either way!

Do you advertise?
Right now I am not advertising very much at all as I have no time to add any new clients to my schedule. The website has been a good marketing tool, and talking about animal rehab at my human practice has been effective as well. My current clients tend to be an excellent source of referrals.

What can you tell us about your successes and struggles?
I think where I have been successful is in my willingness to accommodate to client schedules (i.e. home visits, especially for the geriatric animals). As well, working with the clients to find rehab solutions that fit their lifestyle and budget has been appreciated. From a practice standpoint, I use most of my human physiotherapy education, such as myofascial release, craniosacral, and acupuncture, in my animal practice. These skills have been very useful for me.

I struggle with finding the time to treat more animals. I still need the human hours to pay the bills!

Do you have thoughts on why some rehab facilities fail?
I think that in many cases, the overhead is too high, and therefore, treatment costs have to be too high as well. Both of the failed facilities that I worked with in Edmonton struggled to keep rehab staff, which affected consistency of client care. One facility added charges for every aspect of treatment, which frustrated

clients as they often felt they were being manipulated into getting treatments that they didn't need.

Would you have done anything different?

I would have been more organized with my web site, business cards, etc. I might have looked at hiring someone part time in my human clinic in order to be able to spend more time developing my animal practice more quickly.

Treating animals is often the best part of my day! When I have been frustrated by the human patients, it is nice to go and treat an animal that is happy to see me and actually wants to do their exercises.

Comment on education in the field and what you do to keep current

I think that the learning opportunities in animal rehab have certainly improved over the years, but there is still a lot of room for improvement. Education needs to be easily accessible and affordable. On-line resources would be great!

I try to attend courses and seminars, read articles, and comment threads on the various animal-rehab chat groups. It's hard because it is not easy to get to the courses that are offered. My next step is to increase the time I am able to work with animals and investigate the possibility of getting my master's degree.

Your vision for animal rehab

The future is friendly. At some point, rehab will be an integral part of the care plan for most animals, as it is in human healthcare. There will be multi-disciplinary centres, and there will be stand-alone PT clinics for animals just as there are for humans.

Advice for those just starting out

Just start. Do as much as you can in the time that you have available. Don't be afraid of the challenging cases. They are no different from any challenging human case, and realize that there is always someone to ask for help or suggestions.

Elena Saltis,

NZ Physiotherapist, CCRT
Animal PhysioNZ
Christchurch, New Zealand
www.animalphysionz.com
E-mail: elena@animalphysionz.com
Phone +64 021532672

How did you get started, Elena?

It all started with a small animal physiotherapy course and internship in Australia. I had a dog with wobbler's syndrome and I was treating her myself out of desperation. At the time, my vet built a new building with me in mind and told me to "get my act together and become an animal physio"—so I did! After my course in Australia I was hooked and needed formal education, which is where CRI (The Canine Rehab Institute) came in.

Tell us about you current practice?

I work 90% of the time in the Vet Specialist clinic—the only specialist clinic in the South Island. The caseload breaks down to be approximately 50% ortho, 30% neuro, 10% racing greyhound injury and prevention, and 10% fitness or injury rehab for search and rescue dogs. I see about 40-50 patients a week, and at this time, I am on my own in the rehab department.

Most of my clients are referred to me by Vetspecs, the specialist practice where I work. I am lucky that they refer almost all of their cases to me! I go out to the greyhound-racing kennel each week as well. The urban search and rescue veterinarian refers directly to me, and I also get GP referrals. The referrals are typically emailed to me by the veterinarians, although some GPs phone me up. I get the odd patient through word of mouth or through my website. Once they are in rehab, I treat them in the vet clinic and send out reports to the referring vet's via the vet medical software programme.

What do you do for advertising?

I have brochures in the specialist clinic and also at some vet clinics. I think I have a really cool website, too! I have also given presentations for vet groups and individual in-services for different clinics. The best thing I have found to do is to have a good long chat with the veterinarians directly; I attend veterinary conferences, and during lunch or dinner, talk to them about what I do. Another great tactic I did once was to invite a veterinarian into the airport VIP lounge after an Australian conference and we talked for hours; now he sends me heaps of patients and he is very supportive. I also try to spend time with my specialists, watching surgeries and consults, and I always go to the social events. I think I do my best work at social events, all relaxed! The presentations are nerve racking, and I almost died before a presentation I gave to 80 veterinarians once. Everything has worked out for me, and I don't need to advertise at all, as I can't keep up!

Why do you think that you have been successful?

I believe that what I do is a huge benefit to the animals. I am very dedicated and give it my all. I am confident in my presentation, but at the same time genuinely caring for the animal.

My key to success is the support I have from the specialists. If I relied on GPs I would not be where I am. I was so fortunate that I was able to work myself into Vetspecs, and they wanted a physio and were delighted when I knocked on their door. Luck has been on my side in this arena as well. I also have a good business background. I know how to rebook my patients in for ongoing treatment. The key to that is to believe in what you do.

My over 20 years' experience as a human physio just seemed to translate easily into my animal rehab. It all came very naturally for me. I believe I spent the 20 years practicing on humans to prepare me for the real thing—animals!

How do you keep current?
I keep traveling to the USA to CRI courses! I also go to vet conferences, and the Australian physio society has an animal SIG, so I go to their conferences as well.

My next educational pursuit will be regarding orthotics and prosthetics. My orthopedic surgeon is going with me to the Australia course on this topic, and we are planning on getting into this area of practice together.

What has been your greatest challenge?
In the beginning, trying to juggle owning and operating four large human physiotherapy practices while at the same time working in the vet clinics—it nearly killed me! Since I have sold my human physiotherapy practices, and I am only practicing in the vet clinics, life is better. The earthquake in Christchurch was a big challenge and very stressful, although it did bring in heaps and heaps of patients. Currently, my greatest struggle is trying to fit all the patients into the workweek.

Is there anything else you would like to add?
I think to make this area of practice really work, you need to have full support from at least one specialist orthopedic surgeon. As well, in the future I would like for animal physiotherapy to

become recognized by the New Zealand Physiotherapy Society as a special interest group.

The training I received at CRI, especially from Laurie, was invaluable. (*Editor's note: Elena was not paid or solicited to make this comment!*) CRI made the learning process and retention of information and skills readily accessible. I came out of the courses feeling confident in almost everything I learned; it was incredible. I am so grateful to CRI and the course instructors.

Evelyn Orenbuch,

DVM, CAVCA, CCRT, CVA (candidate)
Georgia Veterinary Rehabilitation,
Fitness & Pain Management (GVR)
Marietta, Georgia, USA
www.GaVetRehab.com
Phone: (678) 803-2626

How did your rehab career start?

I had been practicing veterinary medicine since 1994. In 1998-99, I took the chiropractic classes, but I wasn't comfortable integrating it into my general practice for a while (veterinarians are not taught to do good gentle palpation). Eventually, I started doing more of the chiropractic when one of my co-workers needed her agility dogs worked on. That was a turning point. The adjustments made an incredible difference. I wasn't enjoying my work as a vet associate at the time and saw chiropractic as an opportunity to get out. In January of 2003, I made myself available to do chiropractic at local vet hospitals and for house or stable calls, and I did some relief work. I was seeing quite a few horses at the time. The chiropractic took off so well that I was able to cut back on relief work. In December of 2003, I started the IVAS acupuncture course and completed it by March 2004. During that time, I learned about rehab through one of my clients who had taken her dog out to Chicago to see Dr. Laurie McCauley at Tops Veterinary Rehabilitation, the first purpose-built canine rehabilitation facility. Laurie was the person who suggested I take the acupuncture course. Also on Laurie's suggestion, I then went on to take the canine rehabilitation course at CRI (Canine Rehab Institute). Their course was quite new at that point. I started it at the end of 2004 and finished very early in 2005.

I met the person I thought would be my business partner in the acupuncture class. We took the rehab class together and then packed up a car in February 2005 to drive up and down the east coast visiting different rehab locations and doing a little research to see what everyone was doing at the time. It was eye opening, and that was the beginning of the dream. We wrote a business plan and started looking for locations.

Unfortunately, it didn't work out for the two of us. She followed her boyfriend to Cleveland, leaving me to try to do it on my own, but I didn't feel ready to go brick-and-mortar. Instead, I continued to build my mobile practice. I had a regular route of vet clinics, boarding facilities and agility training barns where I saw patients from New York to Philadelphia. The practice grew and thrived, but it still wasn't the state-of-the-art rehab facility I had always wanted. It took me another five years and a move to Georgia to actualize the dream. I found a new partner, Dr. Alan Cross, who is a board certified surgeon, and we built the first stand-alone rehab facility in Georgia.

Tell me more about the practice
It is a rehab-only private practice. Our caseload consists of approximately 35% neurologic (some of these are old-dog neuro that have osteoarthritis [OA] as well), 20% geriatric/OA, 15% fitness/conditioning, and 30% orthopedic. We usually have over 150 appointments scheduled for any given week. Of course, some of those patients are coming in two to three times in the week, but most are not. Maybe one-third to one-half comes in more than one time per week. We employ, as of October 2013, two full time vets; one part time vet; one part time PT; one full time rehab technician; and three vet assistants/technicians.

Clients come in via referral from primary care or specialty veterinarians, word of mouth, or find us via the internet. Since my business partner is still a partner and surgeon at the largest referral center in Atlanta (Georgia Veterinary Specialists, Blue Pearl), we receive a large number of referrals coming to us from the whole group of specialists. We do a considerable amount of chiropractic, acupuncture and laser, so that is often part of the initial evaluation and re-evaluations. We talk a lot about maintenance and the need to keep coming, even if it is every two to three months to make sure the animal is still doing well and is not developing any new complications or compensations. If in-clinic rehab is needed, we will recommend that they come in one to three times a week to see the therapist, more if it is a neuro case that needs it. We do allow drop offs, but most people don't choose that. Atlanta area traffic is so bad that it simply isn't an option for most people. It would take them twice as long to drive to us, drop off, go to work and then come back. We are near some good shopping though, so on occasion, people choose that as a way to pass time when their animal is in therapy. In most cases, we like to include the owners in the rehab so that they can be a part of the animal's healing, and we feel it makes them more compliant with their exercises at home. So, most people like to stay and help out by offering treats or whatever is needed. Re-evaluations are done every one to three weeks in the beginning, and they then get progressively less frequent, depending on the condition. Billing is done by service, but pre-paid packages are also available.

Tell me about your advertising
We are currently relying primarily on word of mouth from satisfied clients and referring DVMs. We do use social media, and our website is a good source for new clients. I marketed directly to the state veterinary association upon our launch to create

awareness. "Pet fairs" don't seem to give us much return on investment in terms of time spent at the event versus the number of clients acquired. Private workshops and talks to breed and other canine clubs have proved somewhat beneficial. However, the best has been my ability to get up and speak at local CE meetings. Two were sponsored by Georgia Vet Specialists, and they drew a large crowd of local veterinarians from all around the Atlanta area; a third was at the local county VMA. They have a dinner and a CE meeting monthly most of the year. We saw a clear spike in new referrals after each of these speaking opportunities. I like to believe it is because they see that we know what we are talking about, we aren't trying to steal their clients, and our goal is for them to look better because their patients are getting better.

What have been your strengths in making your rehab practice successful?
Strong leadership in terms of our clinic being led by a skilled, experienced rehab veterinary staff, who can offer acupuncture and chiropractic along with the rehabilitation as part of the pain management. There are a few other facilities that offer rehabilitation in our area, but not as their sole focus. We have very high standards for our evaluations and our process. The clients clearly see it every step of the way, from the moment they walk in our door through each appointment. I also think having good business skills is key. I am lucky enough to have a husband who is a business strategist and can help guide us.

What are your thoughts on continuing education in the field, and where you look to upgrade your skills?
The international meetings have been pretty basic. CRI offers very good classes. I can't speak too much of what NES (Northeast Seminars) is doing, but most of my staff was trained there for

their basic certification. I know Healing Oasis has great chiro-practic courses, and my guess is that their rehab is very good as well. We are finally seeing more post-certification courses. The AARV has been holding CE courses at the NAVC meeting in Flori-da for the past several years, but some of that has had to be basic in order to appeal to a larger audience. The STAAR program of-fered in NJ has begun to step things up, and next year, AARV will be working along with them to create an even more advanced track. I'm pleased to see that Rehabilitation and Sports Medicine is a board certification. One of the things that has been lacking is specific, real world studies. With the new board certification, we will be seeing more research in the area. It will be interesting to see where this takes the field.

In addition, I keep current by talking to colleagues (including my PT, who has been a great source of information), and reading the list-serve. In regard to future goals, I would like to be published and then try for the board certification.

Why do you think that some rehab facilities fail?
1) They are run by a tech and not a rehab veterinarian or PT; 2) They do not include chiro and acupuncture (I think these are critical; they allow you to do ongoing treatment as well as treat cases that don't need intense rehab); 3) Poor business practices; 4) Being part of a general practice. It is difficult to market only one part of your hospital. Vets are also inherently nervous about referring to a clinic to which they might lose their patient. 5) Poor skills by the rehab tech or vet. Ultimately, you still have to know what you are doing. You have to be able to correctly diag-nose the problem and know the best solution. 6) Not charging enough.

What has been your greatest struggle?

One challenge has been hiring qualified staff, including veterinarians trained in acupuncture, chiropractic and rehab medicine. We also struggle with balancing "supply and demand"—trying to meet client demand in a timely fashion without diluting the quality of service we offer.

As well, looking back, I would have done some things differently in the creation of my facility. I might have created a more basic space, holding off on some "luxuries" to save money and keep our debt lower.

What would you like to see for the future of animal rehab?

I would like all general practice veterinarians to have an understanding that animal rehabilitation is a serious discipline and that a rehabilitation-certified veterinarian (or possibly a rehab-certified PT) should be overseeing rehab cases. I'd like to see animal rehab become standard of care. When an animal is injured or has surgery or a neurologic issue, the next words out of the primary care or specialist's mouth should be about rehab and how important it is to the improvement of the condition.

Any words of advice?

1) Learn chiropractic and acupuncture; 2) get comfortable with the agility and sport dogs and what they do; 3) give yourself enough room—don't try to work in a tiny space; 4) think big if you want to be big; 5) try not to be a part of an existing clinic unless they are willing to let you spend time marketing and you can do only rehab and not general medicine; 6) you don't need an under-water treadmill to do good rehab.

Helen Nicholson,

BPhty, MAnimSt (Animal Physiotherapy), PhD
Animal Physiotherapy Services
Sydney, New South Wales, Australia
www.k9physio.com - (+61) 2 4739 4557
E-mail: info@k9physio.com

Memberships and Affiliations
Vice-Chair and NSW/ACT of Animal Physiotherapy Group of the Australian Physiotherapy Association

In the beginning…
Back in 1994, while I was studying for my Bachelor of Physiotherapy degree, I saw a picture in a textbook of a snake having physiotherapy for its arthritic spine and I thought, "If it's good enough for a snake, it's good enough for my old Labrador!" So my local vet very kindly encouraged me, explaining to me what was wrong with my dog, asking what I would do if she was a human, explaining to me the relevant anatomy in my dog and asking me to demonstrate the particular technique. He then declared, "That looks safe—go home and do that!" So he and I tackled each of her various diagnoses in the same manner until she died the week before my final exam in November 1996.

After graduating, I had many people approach me for help while I was showing my new dogs. I was aware that there were important differences between the species, and so I waited until I had been able to receive more training before officially beginning my business in 1999.

And your practice now?

My team and I work out of several vet hospitals in the Sydney region and also do tele-rehabilitation sessions for dogs that live too far away to access our services in person. We have four physios, each working "clinic duty" on a part-time basis.

Our caseload is primarily neurological, and orthopaedic (including the geriatric cases). My rough guess is that those types of cases make up 70% of our total caseload. We also see muscular issues and respiratory conditions. I would have no idea about our average weekly case numbers! Last week, we only had one physio on duty, then there was a public holiday and we saw thirty-one cases.

We bill by time, and patients can attend as outpatients, day patients or inpatients for intensive rehab. We can also do tele-rehabilitation via Skype or other means.

How do clients learn about you?

We see patients by vet referral only. We don't advertise at all! However, once or twice a year we send out a newsletter for vet education.

Why do you think that some animal physiotherapy practitioners or facilities/departments fail?

The economics can be precarious. Some services are very expensive to provide, which has to be passed on to the client, and in these economic times, not every client can afford physiotherapy. Other practitioners are also simply not skilled enough, or don't take the extra time that exacting clients require.

What have been your strengths?

Persistence! Demonstrating a commitment to examining animal physiotherapy scientifically (e.g. by doing my PhD) has also really helped build trust with the veterinarians.

Even though my PhD was in animal physiotherapy, what I learnt most was how to monitor and assess the results of treatment from a different perspective. It taught me that things could always be improved upon. So even though my PhD was in a very specific field of animal physiotherapy (i.e. intensive care) I use the skills learnt (e.g. critical thinking, etc.) to help improve my management of every single case.

Struggles? Advice? Your vision for animal physiotherapy

I struggle most with juggling work, study and kids. Persistence can be easier said than done! In fact, looking back I wouldn't have tried to build my business at the same time as having four kids! It's been difficult devoting enough time to both.

I would advise wearing boots so you don't end up with doggy accidents in your socks and to wear thick shirts so cat claws can't get through them easily!

I think the profession will continue to grow, and I would like to see it respected as a specialist field of practice for physiotherapists.

Personally, I am trying to improve my systems so I can better balance my four kids and work. That way, I will have less time taken up with answering emails, for example, so that I have more time to think of new techniques (or drive the kids to sport!).

Anything else?

The variety in animal physiotherapy is much more rewarding than human physiotherapy. My classic example is the day I walked onto a (human) hospital ward to find four post-op cruciate repair patients. Through the open window, we could hear the lifeguards at the neighbouring beach, and it suddenly hit me that there must be more to physiotherapy than protocol-driven monotony! Several years later, I had a day where I treated four dogs following cruciate repair. It struck me how much more enjoyable it was, as even though they were all at the same stage post-operatively and all had the same surgeon, they were all different breeds, had different temperaments, different ages, different willingness to work for food rewards, etc. As a result, I find it much more enjoyable to have to think on my feet every single day, even after all of these years!

Inger Jacobson,

PhD, RPT
Luleå University of Technology
Djursjukhuset Gammelstad
(Animal hospital at Gammelstad, Luleå)
Private practitioner
www.fysorehab.se
inger.jacobson@ltu.se
Luleå, Sweden

Getting started and clinical practice
To start, I simple contacted the local animal hospital, asking if they needed my assistance. I do see some patients in my private practice as well, both canine and equine.

I work full time as a senior lecturer at Luleå University of Technology. Since 2005, I have collaborated with the local animal hospital by assisting them with my knowledge, both in the application of physical therapy to animals, guiding their veterinarians in scientifically writing, as well as developing physiotherapy treatments/guidelines. In return, they teach our animal physiotherapy classes at the university regarding orthopedic examination or acupuncture for dogs.

Inger's animal physiotherapy caseload
I see about 8-12 patients/day, one day/week. Our physiotherapy unit is open four days/week. We have one additional RPT (two days/week) and one rehab nurse (one day/week).

Our local facility cannot accommodate more patients without expanding. We have talked about this for a long time, but we just have to "find the money." I believe we could easily have at least one full-time RPT, one rehab nurse and me (20%), and still be fully booked! This particular animal hospital serves the whole of northern Sweden from Uppsala (900 km south) to the Norwegian/Finnish border in the north (400 km north)! There are other small veterinarian clinics, but no veterinary hospital other than ours in northern Sweden.

It is almost impossible to break down our caseload. We mainly do post-operative rehabilitation (orthopedics), treat overweight patients, provide therapy for back pain, arthritis, or growth diseases (orthopedics), and see some geriatric patients. We seldom provide 'fitness,' as we have so many rehabilitation patients as it is, and we hardly have time for them—maybe in the future!

How Inger practices
Almost all my referrals come from veterinarians at the animal hospital, or from veterinarians in the surrounding geographical areas. I have no need to advertise beyond that!

At the animal hospital, the veterinarians refer the patients to rehab. If the patient has been to rehab recently, they do not need to go to a veterinarian first.

A lot of dogs come to me with a lameness problem. Often, the vet has not seen anything on X-ray and wants me to do a full PT-examination. For treatment, I work with an underwater treadmill. I also utilize exercise balls, balance boards, functional retraining, etc. I am also trained in acupuncture and use it for pain relief. Plenty of time is spent on explaining functional anatomy so that the owner of the dog understands the problem and can come up with additional solutions for home.

In my private practice I always want the patients to have seen a veterinarian first. Most often it is the vet who contacts me and asks me to see the patient. Often in both canine and equine cases it is for an unspecified problem that the vet requests me to examine. I work a lot with acupuncture in dogs as well as with horses.

Since I have worked for over 20 years as a sports medicine RPT (as head of the national under 21 female football team for 8 years, being a clinical sport medicine specialist, and wrote my dissertation in female football injuries), and have trained and competed with German Shepherds (SAR - dog instructor) since 1991, the functionality of the dog is very important to me. Therefore, I place focus on functional training when giving the owners home instructions, and I want to be sure the owners fully understand what to do with their animal and why.

Thoughts on why some animal physiotherapists/facilities fail?

We don't yet have this problem in Sweden. I imagine that it is because rehabilitation can be quite expensive. Each patient takes a lot of time and time costs money. The owner might not be interested in paying so much for the time. In Sweden many dog owners have pet insurance, and there are special rehab-insurances for dogs. That helps!

My biggest struggle has been to get the veterinarians to understand my knowledge and what we can accomplish together as a team. Physiotherapists have so many tools that work with dogs, too. They just need to let us show what we can do!

What are your strengths that have helped you to become successful and what are your continued learning strategies?

My PT-knowledge (sports medicine, orthopedic examination etc.), my human clinical experience, my experience as a dog trainer/handler, and my way of handling the dog-owner has helped me tremendously. You really need to be able to read the dog so that you can see small changes in reactions and subsequently direct your treatment/therapy more specifically. As well, I am an experienced, kind person who genuinely wants to help. I continue to upgrade my knowledge by reading scientific articles, talking to colleagues, going to meetings and conferences, etc.

Visions for the future

I'd like to see RPTs at all veterinary clinics! If you have a veterinarian and a vet nurse, you should have a RPT. There are so many dogs that need our physical therapy skills and knowledge to help them!

My goals are to find MONEY and RPTs that want to be **PhD students** (both in dog and horse scientific projects)! The animal physiotherapy field really needs the backing of science right now to be able to stand up against the veterinarians that still doubt its benefit.

Is there anything you would have done differently when getting started?

"Je ne regret rien," as Edith Piaff said. No, I don't want to change the past.

Words of wisdom

Be humble, but firm. Show what you can do, be proud of this profession. Never stop learning!

Jean C. Pavlakos,

BScPT, CCRP
Our Hearts Canine Rehab
www.ourheartscaninerehab.com
Dayton, Ohio, USA

How it all started for Jean

In high school, my goal was to be a veterinarian. By the time I got to college I decided what I really wanted was an M.R.S. degree and five kids, so I dabbled in a few fields of study and settled on PT as something I could do part time (if at all!) By the time I was 30, I had achieved my MRS, but the five kids were not going to be an option. I revisited vet school, but at that time, the time and financial commitment would leave me in the hole and I would make less as a new vet than I already did as a PT.

By the time I was 45, PT had become a paycheck but not a passion by any sense of the word... I'm not sure it ever was! I changed jobs to see if that would cure my midlife crisis of sorts. The new job was quite a disappointment, except for one of my co-workers who became a dear friend and the conduit to my new profession as a Certified Canine Rehabilitation Practitioner. She had a one-year-old German shepherd with severe hip dysplasia and she was told that the dog needed a hip replacement. This was not in her budget, so her mother went online to pursue other options. They found a woman in our town who had an underwater treadmill (UWTM) for dogs. We all thought this was pretty cool and decided to forgo our usual Thursday night outing (most often a happy hour), and try this thing out! I had a black lab with elbow dysplasia in serious need of some weight loss. It was May, and we went for our first visit. Though interesting, it was not a big success, and we left thinking we would never go back. By November of that year I had been totally unsuccessful in getting my "little fatty" to shed some weight, and I decided to go back for some water exercise. By this time the woman with the treadmill had joined forces with a holistic vet right down the street.

I went weekly, and in casual conversation with the owner/operator of the treadmill (Carmen), she told me that PTs could take classes through the University of Tennessee (UT) to transfer their skills to dogs and that there was already a book out called *Canine Physical Therapy*. Well, that night I ordered the book, obtained the class schedule from UT, and etched out a timeline to complete the program in 1 ½ years. This was it—my dream come true! I could use my PT skills AND work with dogs—without a $40,000 loan.

On Christmas Eve of that year, 2004, as I arrived for my treadmill session, Carmen came running out of the building, hands waving, and shouting, "I have your first patient." Being a planner to a fault, this was not how I had pictured my new venture in my head. I had courses to take and studying to do. But as the saying goes, *No better time than the present.* I agreed to give it a shot. Both Carmen and the vet accepted me unconditionally into their practice and *…the rest is history!*

How Jean practices

I am an outpatient practice, which I own and operate. I am housed in a building with an UWTM, owned and operated by another practitioner and a holistic vet. The vet owns the building, and I rent space from her. I pay all my own expenses—insurance, equipment, upkeep of my space, cleaning, etc. I bill, collect, and schedule all my own patients. Referrals come from the two in-house vets and those that I bring in from the outside.

I still practice part-time human orthopedics and sports medicine, but I am also full-time at practicing in canine rehab. Myself, I average 30 patients a week, and the underwater treadmill sees approximately 30 patients a week. Some of those, perhaps one-half, are patients that we both see. The caseload is made up of 50% orthopedic patients (post-ops and sports injuries), 25% geriatric, and 25% neurologic. The UWTM is approximately the same, with a small fitness group as well. We are essentially three different business housed in one building: one PT (me), an UWTM (administered by an unlicensed vet assistant), and two vets (plus a secretary).

The initial evaluation is one hour, during which time I get a history as the dog is moving about the room getting comfortable (I am also watching how the dog moves). I then do my evaluation, including a gait assessment in the parking lot, a treatment, and creation of a home exercise program (Note: I always have the owners practice the exercises in front of me). They are then given handouts for the exercises and a follow-up e-mail that includes digital pictures of the same. Next, I explain to them what would be the ideal treatment schedule, (i.e. frequency and number of visits). I am very specific with them that our goal is to meet the dog's needs AND their resource ability (i.e. time and money). Together, we develop a plan that accommodates both (which is almost never the ideal). I collect my fee, write a receipt, and schedule their return appointment on the back of my business card. The clients are urged to call or email any questions that come up before the next visit as compared to waiting until the appointment. I think this is especially important for the nervous owners. At home, I type an evaluation summary and send it to all vets involved in the dogs care.

Follow-ups are 30-minute outpatient appointments with the owner in attendance throughout. Only once in seven years have I asked the owner to step out, as it was more distracting for the dog to have her present! I have no assistant, so I engage the owner to help with the exercise (i.e. feeding treats, etc.) The owner becomes involved in the care, sees how the exercises are to be performed, and understands the goals of each element of the treatments. I also find that I learn a lot from the owners as to their dog's behaviors and reactions. I feel the "buy in" to therapy from the owners is greater when they are part of it. During the follow-up sessions, I usually start with a quick evaluation of the target areas, then perform modalities (I only have a laser, actually) and hands-on therapies (my MOST beneficial and cheapest tool!), mobilizations, PNF (proprioceptive neuromuscular facilitation), osteopathy, etc. Progression is made to the exercise portion (i.e. balance board, ball, cavalettis, etc.) and ends with PROM and stretching once the muscles are warmed up. I have a flow sheet for documentation, which is mostly a checklist with room for subjective and objective measurements. Lastly, I collect my fee, provide a receipt, and schedule the next appointment. About half of the dogs I see have either already been in the UWTM or partake in an UWTM session after my treatment. The UWTM is scheduled concurrently but billed separately.

My short-term (by this time next year) goal is to increase my volume to 40 visits/week; right now I am at 30-35. My long-term dream is to have a property with facilities to house dogs for in-patient care.

Finding clients, or rather, clients finding Jean
Presently, most of my referrals come from previous clients (word of mouth), presentations at dog clubs, three specialty centers in a 50-mile radius, and four or five local primary care vets, as well as two in-house holistic vets. Clients will call or email me directly. When I schedule them, I send them a referral form for their vet, and explain my procedures, location and pricing schedule.

In regards to advertising, I have a website, which originally was the primary way owners found me, and then I would have them go to their vets for referrals. I also have brochures, business cards and magnets.

My best marketing strategy by far and away, was to go to local performance events to watch, learn and interact. I wasn't there to sell myself, but to let them know I was interested in learning and understanding the different events and what their dogs were competing in (they don't care how much you know until they know how much you care!) Of course, I always had my business cards on hand! Once I was somewhat well known in that circuit, I started doing a series of seminars for the dog clubs and this increased my referrals even more.

From the start I always sent professionally typed reports with evaluation summaries and progress notes to each surgeon and family vet as well as monthly rehab status reports. These are time consuming, but worth it!

Jean's thoughts on the failure of some rehab facilities and departments:
Communication is critical! I think owner involvement is the key to their "buy–in" to the process and willingness to spend their

time and money. I sometimes answer emails and phone calls until 8 or 9 o'clock at night so that the owners know I am responsive to their needs. I also feel that interacting with **all** of the vets involved in the dogs care is crucial, (i.e. the surgeon as well as the primary vet).

Also, when I started I had an 8-foot x 10-foot space in a vet clinic and one ball I dusted off from a long forgotten home exercise plan for myself. I cleaned the clinic weekly to offset my rent. I only added equipment and then space when my business had grown and only purchased equipment that I had saved for. I will say, the first year of my education was financed out of my personal savings, but after that, I paid as I went. I have always maintained hours at my human job to supplement my income but have gradually decreased those hours as my canine rehab business grew. Bottom line is, I didn't invest in a lot before I knew I had the business to support it!

Jean's strengths and how she has enhanced her skills and knowledge

I absolutely LOVE the dogs, all of them, even the ones that bite me (though there has only been a couple of the latter). I think the owners and the dogs sense this love and know that I will do everything in my power to help them. I have also made continued learning a priority: reading, seminars, and going to performance events.

I think my sports medicine background has helped me a lot, especially with the performance dogs. In particular, looking at exercise from a functional and closed-chain perspective, since dogs do most everything closed-chain. In choosing my continuing education courses required for my human PT license, I look for courses that will carry over to my canine clients.

I try to take at least two continuing education courses or seminars each year (i.e. University of Tennessee, the Canine Rehab Institute, Therapaw, Patricia Kortekaas, and the international vet-rehab symposium). I subscribe to Clean Run magazine, the American Canine Sports Medicine Association, Wizard of Paws, and the Whole Dog Journal. I also order videos and books (I especially like Debbie Gross Saunders video's and Chris Zink's books). The Vet-Rehab list-serve is very valuable and I subscribe to a website—iknowlegdenow.com—for research. I have also attended a few dog behavior seminars and presentations through our local vet association.

Jean's advice

1. Physical therapists need a vet referral to practice (in most states), but until the vets see your results they may not buy-in to the need for your skills or service. So, you need patient results to get referrals, but referrals to get patients! You have to work backwards. Go to the source. Get involved with local dog clubs. These people will move heaven and earth to get good treatment for their pups. They will go to their vets and ask for referrals. Then once the dog is a patient of yours, communicate often with the vet and develop the relationship and trust.

2. I also think it is crucial to work with the owners to meet their time and financial resources. Offer alternatives, such as rechecks with a comprehensive home program versus weekly rehab. Once they see the changes, they will ask to come more often. If you overwhelm the client on the first visit, you are sure to lose them! The vets also appreciate a clinician that doesn't oversell their service or appear to only be interested in lining their pockets.

3. Make sure your service is customer friendly. Never forget these owners are choosing to spend what disposable income they have with you. Provide convenient time frames for the clients. Most people work, and they have to, to pay your fee, so offer time slots after work. Most nights I am at the clinic until 7-8 pm. Fees should be reasonable. Though I am long overdue for a rate increase, due to the economic down turn, I have kept my prices lower and my volume has continued to increase.

4. If you get behind, don't shortchange a client to catch up. I worked with an orthopedic surgeon who taught me a very valuable lesson. He used to say, "The later I am, the more behind I get." His point being that, if people have to wait, they start to get aggravated, so make sure when they leave that they felt that they got their money's worth and that you were worth waiting for!

Jean's views on the future of animal rehab

Years ago, human physical therapy was considered risky and not well understood. For example, back surgeons told their patients, go home, rest, and just walk... in dog terms—cage rest! Then, back patients were sent for hot packs, ultrasound, massage... but God-forbid, no exercise! Now, back patients are sent primarily and expediently to Rehab. Some insurance companies won't even pay for an MRI without first trying PT. So, I see veterinary medicine going in the same direction. As vets and the public understand better what we do, Rehab will become the norm.

I would also like to see physical therapists included in all state veterinary practice acts. Ohio just added PTs to theirs. Presently, however, a vet must be on-site for us to treat. I would like to see a provision for PT's to operate independently of the vet (with a written referral), if they have completed and passed a certification program.

Final words of wisdom

The only regret I have is that I didn't find this sooner in my career; however, I truly believe God didn't send me this opportunity until I was ready for it.

One additional thing I believe has been my secret weapon: Each day before I start treatment I say a silent prayer as follows, "Dear Lord, please give me the strength, knowledge and focus I need to treat your sweet angels. In your name I deliver their care,".... He has never let me down! ☺

Jennifer Gordon,

BScPT, CCRT, CAFCI
The Canine Fitness Centre
Calgary Alberta, Canada
jenn@caninefitness. com
www. caninefitness. com

Jennifer's beginnings:

I started practicing Canine Rehab in 2008, but before that, around 2004, I subscribed to CPA's CHAP newsletter—Canadian Horse and Animal Physiotherapy Association—now the Animal Rehab Division of the CPA. I loved reading about the canine conditions and the work physiotherapists were doing in that field. I remember reading about a makeshift "door" wobble board for a Great Dane and I thought that was brilliant! How exciting to be involved in a growing field of physiotherapy with animals I loved. At that time I was still learning and growing in my human profession, but I realized that much of what I was learning was applicable to the canine skeleton—manual therapy skills, exercises, body mechanics and muscle imbalances had similar principles. Hmmm, maybe I could do both!

I took my first course in 2006, the Animal Rehab Division's Introduction to Canine Rehab. While learning the anatomy and canine conditions were a challenge, I found I had a good understanding of the manual techniques and assessment/treatment principles. I was intrigued at this new challenge and began shadowing the therapists at the Canine Fitness Centre. I was soon encouraged to enroll in the Canine Rehabilitation Institutes program and attain my Certified Canine Rehab Therapist (CCRT) qualification. I completed my Introduction to Canine Rehab and The Canine Rehab Therapist modules in 2008. In the spring of 2009, I completed the Canine Sports Medicine module and achieved my designation of CCRT.

Jennifer's practice:
I have had the fortune of working at the Canine Fitness Centre, a stand-alone rehabilitation clinic for dogs, and I am continuing to learn and be challenged with each case I see! It is a fascinating field and it is a joy to be involved in an aspect of the physiotherapy profession that is breaking ground in both research and recognition.

The therapists there are both physiotherapists and CCRTs. We have four Physiotherapists/CCRTs and three assistants and as clinic we see 40-60 clients per week. As a practitioner, I work once a week at this clinic and see approximately 3-5 clients per week, predominately orthopedic cases—approximately 70%—the remaining make up Fitness/Conditioning at 10%, Geriatric at 10%, and finally Neuro at 10%.

We bill by time allotments for both physiotherapy and underwater treadmill sessions. We do require a vet referral for rehab cases at our clinic, so a client is typically referred to us by their vet. If they come to our clinic on their own accord, we will contact their vet for medical records, etc. So once they're "in" they may have rehab therapy, underwater treadmill therapy, neuromuscular training, modalities, or fitness conditioning, depending on what is appropriate. Interestingly, our referrals are roughly 50% from primary DVMs and 50% owner requests. There is a mix in there from specialty vets, such as surgeons that refer to our clinic.

We mainly advertise directly to the primary DVMs through a newsletter. We market through social media with a website and facebook page. The owners give talks at the U of Calgary Faculty of Vet Medicine, and have on occasion given talks for local Calgary media. Word of mouth through clients at dog shows and competitions is probably our best advertisement!

Jennifer's strengths as a Canine Rehab Therapist:

I think my manual therapy skills from physiotherapy have helped me with my hands on skills with canine patients. I have taken advanced courses in manual therapy and feel this helps me have a better sense of muscle tone, joint play, joint mechanics and physical abnormalities that I can transfer to the canine patient. I also relate well with people, and (most!) dogs, and hopefully, this has helped owners and clients feel at ease with me personally and with my expertise as a therapist.

We also discuss cases and techniques among the therapists at our clinic, I read notes/textbooks from the courses I have taken and I have subscribed to an online learning resource with current research, video training and links to discussion groups/further resources/etc. (i.e. Four Leg Rehab!).

Struggles and challenges are a part of the business:

Most dogs are great to treat, but the occasional dog that doesn't want to sit or lay down for assessment is a challenge! I feel like I don't get an adequate assessment with some of these clients. Another challenge is learning what is typical for dogs healing from certain injuries or conditions. As I have not been practicing for long in this field, I don't have the experience under my belt to be confident with certain scenarios.

Some rehab businesses fail if they do not establish good working relationships with referring vets. Communication and collaboration are very important! I think our facility excels with the help of our large fitness/conditioning area. If a rehab facility does not have the right environment to cater to canine clients they may not have longevity with their clientele.

What does the future hold for Canine Rehab and Jennifer?

The ARD has quite a good course outline, including home study, Intro and Advanced courses. These are very informative and hands on courses. The CRI in the US has an extensive course program as well, with many options for further studies beyond the certification program. I feel there are many options to learn and update your knowledge. For us Canadians, the CRI courses involve extensive travel expenses on top of the tuition. This can be a limiting factor for many therapists here. As the profession grows and the demand for more courses increases, I hope for some "tune up" courses that may focus on certain conditions commonly treated or fitness/conditioning/exercise ideas, for example.

I do see this field growing and becoming more recognized. As it grows there are many "practitioners" jumping on the rehab bandwagon, and I hope that we can protect our expertise of physiotherapy with this population. This is important for the safety of our canine clients as well as for the protection of our profession. We cannot let other canine caregivers simply say they do "rehab" without the expertise that we offer. I hope that more vets become knowledgeable in what we have to offer and this field becomes more collaborative. I think the limitation in this area has to do with primary DVMs and specialty vets not understanding our expertise and knowledge base.

Personally, I would love to take the Canine Neurological Rehab Course offered by the CRI or an equivalent course from the ARD and learn more in that area. I would be interested in assisting the instruction of the ARD certification courses, as the best way to know a skill is to teach others! Attending some agility and sporting events would also benefit my practice in giving me a greater understanding of the body mechanics and challenges these canine athletes experience.

With that being said, I would recommend attending agility events, dog shows, canine sporting competitions, and shadowing in both a vet and a physiotherapy setting. Looking back, I think shadowing in a vet clinic would've helped me understand different conditions, surgical procedures and protocols on that end. This is also something I could do currently as a learning opportunity!

Jim Berry,

BSc, MSc, DVM
Douglas Animal Hospital
Fredericton, NB, Canada
E-mail: Jberry59@gmail.com
Phone: 506-458-5944

How did you get started, Jim?

I was already doing acupuncture and massage, so it was a natural fit to start to incorporate rehab. I took my training through the Canine Rehab Institute in 2006, and I think that the best part of it all, from my perspective, was the diagnostic techniques that rehab added to my practice. Vet practice treats lameness as a joint, bone, or soft tissue issue. Rehab expands upon this, especially the soft tissue aspects. Thus, I found that it opened up the possibility of specific diagnoses and treatments for lameness. It allowed me to start utilizing stretches, strengthening exercises, and laser, as well as start to really target post-operative rehabilitation for orthopaedic cases.

How does rehab fit into your practice?

I work out of a clinical veterinary office. I see approximately five rehab cases a week. 75% of those are orthopaedic, 15% are geriatric, and the rest are mainly conditioning. Most clients are either my own clients already (50%) or are referred by other local vets for refractory pain, etc. (50%).

Rehab depends a lot on the individual case, but it is often structured as one to two visits per week after the initial assessment. We send clients home with written information on exercises, stretches, etc. as a home program to be carried out between sessions. My technicians often perform the laser treatments, and I do the acupuncture. We usually charge by prepaid package for laser and acupuncture and charge by time for diagnosis and physical manipulations.

Your strengths

I incorporate some elements of rehab in every case I see, from routine physical exams for vaccines to lameness or geriatric work ups. I also try to keep things very simple. I really enjoy physical/hands-on manipulation, and subsequently, I do not use a lot of equipment (except the laser). This allows me to use a lot of rehab techniques and keep the cost reasonable, with good owner compliance.

I used to use acupuncture as a separate part of practice. Now I often have patients receiving laser, acupuncture, stretching, and weight loss programs concurrently. I rarely fragment what I do now.

Can you comment on education in the field?

I find that I struggle with finding the time to learn more. I mainly try to find information and education online. I do try to get continuing education in canine rehab, but that is difficult at this point in time.

Most of the courses are either in the US or seem to be in places that are too hard to get to from the Atlantic Provinces in Canada. To fly anywhere, I need to go through Toronto or Montreal, so travel takes a lot of time. I would like to see good quality on-line continuing education. I am hoping to certify in pain management in the next year and then take some advanced courses in physical manipulation techniques.

Your vision for the future of animal rehab

Rehabilitation is starting to gain wide acceptance in the veterinary world. Ideally, I would like to see basic rehab courses brought into the vet school curriculum so all new graduates could do basic rehab on their own orthopaedic, lame, or geriatric patients and know when to refer to specialists.

Advice

Start slow. Use your hands and your judgment, and leave the toys for later when you know if you really need them and can make them pay their way.

Julia Tomlinson,

BVSc, MSc, PhD, DAVCS, CCRP, CVSMT
Twin Cities Animal Rehabilitation Clinic
Twin Cities metro, Minnesota, USA
www.tcrehab.com
E-mail: drjulia@tcrehab.com

Julia's background

I started with a BVSc, then went on to obtain a Masters in ultra-sonographic versus MRI anatomy of the equine pelvis, finished up with a PhD on NSAIDs. I obtained my DAVCS status in equine surgery and practiced as an equine surgeon at NC State and MS State from 2001-2005. My greatest interest was in lameness and sports medicine.

I became injured as the result of three separate incidences—once during my residency by a horse, and then in two separate car accidents. I struggled physically to work with horses (e.g. flexion tests, and lifting), and I was in a lot of chronic pain. Subsequently, I sought help from many different sources: MD, PT, chiropractor, Carrick neurologist (who helped the most), sports rehabilitation, acupuncture, energy work, and homeopathy. Each of these therapeutic choices was focused on for a period of time before I moved to the next and each helped to varying degrees (apart from the MD who said I had chest wall syndrome, common in women, and to try anti-depressants. I only managed to convince her I was in pain when I showed her a pain diary I had kept!). All of these experiences contributed to my interest in rehabilitation and chronic pain management. I realized there are very few practitioners out there who effectively advocate for their patients, who can coordinate care with a team approach and who will not give up on a case, even if they cannot help the patient themselves—they will work to find someone who can.

Once I realized I could no longer be an equine sports medicine veterinarian, I researched other career paths. It was a pretty low point in my life. I had completed my PhD after my residency and had realized that research, although interesting, isolated me from patients and was not for me. A close friend had given up being an equine surgeon for different reasons and had retrained as a small animal surgeon. She helped to mentor me through my career "crisis," and suggested small animal rehabilitation as a career path. I was curious enough to shadow a rehabilitation veterinarian, Dr. John Sherman, in North Carolina. He helped me to understand how much I could bring from my old career and who to talk to and train with in order to change paths. I spent time working in small animal emergency medicine to provide myself an income. At the same point in time, I shadowed a small animal surgeon, did externships at rehabilitation practices when I could, pursued my CCRP certification (2006), and also shadowed in a regular vet practice. I re-read textbooks from my vet school days and read newer texts in sports medicine and rehabilitation.

Dr. John Sherman helped me with a business model to open my own rehabilitation practice, and we opened in 2007. I have continued my training and also obtained my CVSMT in 2009. Canine rehabilitation is the most rewarding job I have ever had. I hesitate to call it a job. It is a vocation that suits me perfectly!

The practice
I practice in a stand-alone clinic that was customized within a 2500 square foot space. I see an average of 14 cases per day. Ad-

ditional cases are seen for therapies provided by the staff and my other veterinarian who currently works two days a week alongside me. The caseload consists of 5% conditioning and fitness (which increases during the winter months), 25% geriatric, 15% neuro, 55% ortho (mix of post op and non-surgical, but only 20% are post op). The overall caseload is 45% sporting dogs. The practice consists of two rehabilitation vets (one currently part-time), one rehabilitation tech, one tech student, and one assistant. I also have contract workers—a massage therapist and an acupuncturist.

Clients often seek out our services directly, but more and more veterinary referrals are occurring now (we are in our fifth year of business presently). It seems that once a client finds us, they report back to their vet and then their vet sends us more cases. The surgeons still only refer the problem cases, or "soft tissue" cases that they want me to diagnose. We get very little routine post-op. The sporting dog community is very tight knit, and I am well known there, however. 50% of our cases come by vet referral and the other 50% find us on their own.

The rehabilitation program(s): Initial examinations are done by myself or other veterinarian with me overseeing (she is a recent CCRP and I am a control freak—no surprise there!). The initial plan is devised and the client is educated that the plan will change according to progress. We do daily rounds to discuss the plan for therapies that day, which gives us time to discuss progress and troubleshoot, etc., as necessary. Homework usually changes weekly, not at every visit. Pain management is very important as well and the vets manage this aspect, but the techs contribute to the pain assessment. We also provide "home" plans and check in frequently. Manual therapies are very important at my clinic and an integral part of management of every case.

Our advertising is primarily word of mouth, and we do have a website as well. Our least successful strategy has been advertising in the VMA newsletter.

Julia's strengths

Tenacity, both in business and with my patients, has helped me tremendously. As well, I feel that I provide the support that people cannot get elsewhere, and I am constantly an advocate for the patient and client, even with regular veterinary issues. I can help to see the global picture (usually). Spending additional time to educate the client and referring vets about the condition the patient has also serves me well.

My skills as an equine diagnostician aid me. I use flexion tests, stress tests, and sometimes even diagnostic anesthesia. I think palpation skills are more developed in equine practitioners. I also use ultrasound to diagnose (using my equine skills and an anatomy book!) and I am working on growing that skill. Knowledge of surgical procedures and biomechanics helps, as does thinking outside the box—you have to as an equine clinician. My skills as a "chiropractor" I use on almost every case, and also needle trigger point therapy. Lastly, I incorporate making or modifying assistive devices into my practice.

The failure of some rehabilitation practitioners or facilities

I think that some people/practices fail because they don't charge enough to cover their costs; they don't commit trained personnel to it full time; they subsidize with money from other services, and they don't "sell" their value. I am really concerned about regular vets and techs offering "rehabilitation" that is not practiced to any real skill level; it is downgrading the discipline. The rehabilitation certification courses are just the beginning and those certified vary hugely in skill set (I don't mean to sound like a snob). However, this can turn clients away from rehabilitation altogether, as they do not get the results they sought.

Keeping current and Future plans

I LOVE the New Jersey Therapaw seminar, and I love my chiropractic continuing education, as there is so much functional neurology training. My knowledge is additionally furthered by attending continuing education lectures and reading journals. With the AARV *[American Association of Rehabilitation Practitioners]*, we have been so busy introducing rehabilitation to newbies that we don't get enough advanced info; the Therapaw seminars help with that. More advanced information is definitely needed.

My next plans are to complete my ACVSMR boards and then to move to a bigger space. I'd like to try delegating more of the business aspects of my practice as well.

Struggles and hopes for the future of animal rehabilitation

As we get busier, devoting enough time to the thought process about managing each case becomes difficult. It is easy to get onto automatic pilot.

I would love to see the more people take on becoming ACVSMR board certified and for rehabilitation to become a fully integrated part of veterinary care, for it to become the "norm" as part of case management is perhaps a better way to put it.

Advice

Commit to it, but have a backup source of income! (I taught vet techs and did emergency work part time during the first nine months we were open.) Provide the opening hours that clients need to get to you—and your location should be easy access, but it does not need to be prominent (AKA expensive rent).

Julie Mayer,

DVM, CVA, CVC, CCRP
Integrative Veterinarian
Phoenix, Arizona, USA
www. integrativeveterinarian.com
dr. julie@integrativeveterinarian.com
Cell: 312-405-6444

How Julie got started

I became certified in veterinary acupuncture in 1996 and started my own house call business, Healing Arts For Animals. As I was developing my skills and learning acupuncture methods and its benefits, I realized that the chronic arthritis and chronic lame patients' pain was resolving with acupuncture, but the needles could not move the subluxations in the joints. So, off to get certified in veterinary chiropractic I went! My chiropractic skills and knowledge definitely were the segue into the rehab world. I was able to diagnose and treat many injuries, chronic musculoskeletal issues, age related problems, neurological situations, and more. When I would adjust animals, I would instruct the client to perform therapeutic exercises to correct abnormalities that preceded the problem in order to prevent a recurrence. I also used ultrasound quite frequently for tendinitis and other soft tissue injuries. I used a lot of electroacupuncture and TENS for pain management, post-operatively and in acute situations. When I started there were no rehabilitation certification courses available, so I read several human and equine texts and learned the different interventions and modalities available at that time. I also did some agility with my Rat Terrier and attended many canine sports events. In 2000, I became the Director of Therapet, a new rehab facility at the Veterinary Specialty Center in Illinois. After working at Therapet for several years, I co-founded and opened a stand-alone 6000 square foot rehab, holistic, and wellness center in Chicago. Presently, I am in Arizona practicing rehabilitation, sports medicine, and holistic veterinary medicine.

What does your practice look like now?
Right now I am an independent contractor in Arizona and work at three different locations and do house calls. Two locations are veterinary hospitals that have rehab departments in their clinics, and the other location is an indoor dog gym and training facility where I have an office and can see patients. I am also preparing to open up a rehabilitation and sports medicine center with a Board Certified Orthopedic Surgeon.

On average, I see approximately 50 cases a week. 50% are sports and soft tissue injury, 30% are post-op/orthopedic, 10% are senior dogs (arthritis, degenerative neuropathy, pain management, etc.), 5% are neurologic, and the remaining 5% is comprised of fitness and conditioning.

The sequence of events for patients engaging our services: DVMs +/- PTs together do the initial evaluation and design the protocol on the first visit. The DVM sends out a referral report to the referring hospital and occasionally calls the referring vet. The modalities are executed by rehab certified therapists or the PTs and occasionally the DVM. The DVM +/- PT reevaluates the patient (i. e. checks measurements, gait, neuro, etc.) every two to three weeks or so throughout the program. There is an exit exam with the DVM +/- PT, at which point the client is encouraged to join membership and continue fitness/wellness/conditioning/tune-ups. The DVMs perform the acupuncture and the chiropractic as prescribed in the protocol. The DVM sends out the final referral report.

Where do your referrals come from and how do you advertise?

With the referrals in order of most to least, they come from pet owner, general practitioners/primary care DVMs, pet professionals (dog walkers, groomers, trainers, etc.), and then veterinary surgeons.

My advertising is comprised of "word of mouth," social media (website, blog, Facebook, Twitter, and My Space), having a booth or volunteering at community events (5k runs for example), speaking engagements (breed, agility clubs, veterinarian continuing education lectures, vet schools, etc.), rehab certification websites, brochures/business cards (via mail to the general practitioners), and personally attend sporting events.

Why do you think that some rehab facilities or departments fail and what have been your strengths?

I think that some rehab practices fail because they are not staffed properly (i. e. with qualified personnel) and they do not have or devote enough time to the rehab department. I have also found it to be difficult to get orthopedic surgeons and neurologists to refer. Additionally, I feel that rehab centers should devote more of a focus on rehab for obese and overweight pets, since they are more than 50% of our caseload.

For over 12 years I have devoted my veterinary career to holistic medicine and rehabilitation. That is all I do! I believe that I have better outcomes and results because I combine the acupuncture and chiropractic skills that I have acquired. As well, I have always paid attention to detail and make sure that I can give the best quality of care and service possible.

Do you have any advice for other starting out in this field?
You have to promote both yourself and this discipline. Reach out and approach veterinary hospitals and give presentations on your services and case studies. Host seminars and CE events at your facility. Get out into the community and attend animal-related sporting events. Learn how animals move and study anatomy. The better a practitioner and diagnostician you are, the better you can serve your patients, which leads to better out-comes and a great reputation! Those of you who are veterinarians, I would get certified in chiropractic. It really helps to understand the musculoskeletal system. In addition, acupuncture is also a great tool for pain management.

Any further comments?
Acupuncture helps me tremendously with treating pain and neurological diseases and deficiencies. Chiropractic is definitely beneficial to the rehab patient by treating primary and compensatory issues, which hastens recovery. Knowledge in nutrition and nutraceuticals can help the patients heal quicker and support the body for the long term. I think that more information on nutrition should be incorporated into rehab protocols. Textbooks are deficient in this area, and I cannot stress how important it is to feed the canine athlete correctly in order to achieve a healthy, injury-free career.

In vet school I wanted to be an orthopedic surgeon. If I would have pursued that path along with these other trades, then I might be better able to show my orthopedic DVM colleagues the necessity of rehab in veterinary medicine. I wish I had finished writing the rehab book that I started very early on in my career!

I look forward to seeking board certification in the future, focusing on public and professional speaking engagements, and designing rehab equipment, materials, and teaching aides. I've had a great journey so far and great opportunities to advance myself in this discipline.

Karen Atlas,

MPT, CCRT

Hydropaws Animal Rehabilitation and Performance Center
Santa Barbara, California, USA
www.hydropaws.com
(805) 687-4131
karen@hydropaws.com

The Inspiration

My life changed after adopting my injured dog, Teddy. I was told by several veterinarians that his lameness would resolve with restricted activity and medications. Unfortunately, he was allergic to the prescribed medications and became very ill. I went to many different veterinarians for second, third and fourth opinions, but none could help my Teddy.

Trained as a human physical therapist, I hoped that I could use my rehabilitation skills to relieve his pain; I knew, though, that I needed specialized training in canine anatomy and biomechanics. I searched the Internet at first with the intention of taking a canine anatomy course just so I could find how I could use some of my human-trained techniques on Teddy. But my search led me much deeper than I anticipated. It was during that time that I learned that certification in canine rehabilitation was possible, and found that the Canine Rehabilitation Institute was a good match for me. I was "all in" after that point.

Canine rehabilitation soon became my passion. Little did I know when I adopted my sweet Teddy that he would completely change my career direction and life (and the lives of many more of his species!). Canine rehab was a perfect fit for me, as it meshed my love for dogs with a profession that I had already been successfully practicing for 12 years.

I was very fortunate to meet a leader in the field of veterinary medicine, Dr. Kenneth Bruecker, Board Certified Veterinary Surgeon. He was looking for a licensed physical therapist with advanced training in canine rehabilitation to lead his new rehab clinic within his highly regarded referral-only specialty hospital, Veterinary Medical and Surgical Group (VMSG). I worked with Dr. Bruecker and developed the new department, eventually leaving his practice to be closer to home following the birth of my first child.

I then teamed up with a local veterinarian, Dr. Dave Dawson, who completed his certification classes and created a canine rehabilitation clinic behind his existing practice, called Hydropaws Animal Rehabilitation and Performance Center. Dr. Dawson was too busy to run both a veterinary hospital and a rehab clinic, and he understood the importance of having a licensed physical therapist trained in canine rehabilitation as part of the team to grow the rehab center. I have been the Director of Hydropaws now for over five years; in addition to patient care, I am responsible for overall management, program development, training, and staffing.

The Practice

Hydropaws is a dedicated rehabilitation facility attached to a well-regarded veterinary hospital. The veterinary hospital has six veterinarians on staff. We have two underwater treadmills, a land treadmill, two class 3B cold laser units, an ultrasound/electrical stimulation combo unit, a portable neuromuscular electrical stimulation (NMES) unit, a portable TENS unit, a pulsed electromagnetic field (PEMF) mat, an Alpha-Stim machine, a treatment table, and a wide range of other equipment, ranging from physioballs, balance discs and wobble boards, to caveletti poles, a ramp, an exercise ladder and stairs.

We have about 45-55 visits each week, with some patients requiring multiple visits. The caseload consists of approximately 70% Ortho, 20% Neuro, and 10% Geriatrics. We employ three aides (one full time and two part-time, at approximately 25-30 hours each), and benefit from the support staff of the adjacent veterinary hospital. As the only therapist, I frequently have waiting lists for new clients.

The Typical Visit
We require a veterinarian referral to begin the rehab process. Once it has been determined that the animal is medically stable to safely undergo rehabilitation, we receive the referral, obtain all medical records, and schedule an initial evaluation.

Upon a patient's first visit, we require intake paperwork, which includes a functional questionnaire (past and present functional abilities and client goals for rehab), and consent forms (right to use photography/video for treatment and marketing purposes, cancellation policy, etc.). Initial appointments require 75-90 minutes, and they include a comprehensive evaluation and treatment for that day. During this time, I am assisted by an aide who helps with animal handling and documents my findings so my focus can remain on the patient and client. After a thorough assessment, I discuss my findings with the client. I then make my recommendations for a treatment plan to reach their specific goals and we schedule additional appointments, as needed. The client leaves with a solid understanding of what their pet is facing and what steps we are going to take to improve their quality of life and reach their goals based on as much evidence-based research as possible. Subsequent sessions then range from 30-75 minutes.

The Marketing Process

When I started at Hydropaws, I developed the logo and marketing materials, including business cards, brochures, educational materials, and small gift items (pens, water bottles, tote bags) to promote our brand. I went to every vet clinic in my area and dropped off my marketing collateral, with the hope of introducing myself and our practice to the veterinarians. I also offered a free staff education in-service visit to each clinic.

Unfortunately, my efforts met a great deal of resistance. Very few vets would give me any time at all, even for a brief introduction, and only one clinic took me up on my offer to do an in-service. It was discouraging to find that very few vets were open to hearing what I had to offer for the benefit of their patients.

But I persevered. I was asked to speak at a local kennel club, which went very well. As patients slowly trickled in, it was my outcomes that soon came to speak for themselves. Clients and vets started to see the dramatic improvements that rehab could bring, and business began to grow. Word of mouth is very important in my small community; I knew that nothing short of excellence would generate the buzz we needed to succeed.

I began attending two of the largest canine public adoption events in town, setting up booths, putting out our equipment, and talking to the festivalgoers about what Hydropaws can offer. I receive terrific feedback at these events, from new people that we educate, to clients who just stop by our booth to say hi and share some smiles and wags.

In the beginning, I also held an open house and brought in a celebrity dog trainer and author, Tamar Geller, who had experienced first-hand the benefits of our services. We offered a meet-and-greet and book signing with Tamar and demonstrated our rehab techniques. Other marketing strategies: Website and Facebook—we post our inspiring patients for the community to see. I get consistent positive feedback from our Facebook page. I found that print ads were not cost effective, as the target market is too narrow for this medium.

Referrals come from specialty hospitals, primary care DVMs (from our affiliated veterinary practice as well as outside vets). Often, clients contact us directly to request rehab; in these cases, we contact the patient's primary DVM to obtain medical clearance before initiating rehab.

The Ingredients for Success

My experience in starting and directing a human physical therapy clinic earlier in my career helped to build Hydropaws into the success it is today. Additionally, strong interpersonal skills are critical to building healthy and trusting relationships within the community (both with vets and clients). And finally, passion for the profession must shine through; my clients sense my genuine effort to help their pets as if they were my own.

The Barriers to Success

In addition to experience, interpersonal skills, and passion, there is no substitute for specialized training. Most clinics that I see fail tend to hire the more economical, but often inadequately trained, person to render professional rehab services. This is not only bad medicine for the patients, but also bad for the profession of canine rehab. Buying the fancy equipment, hanging a sign, and hiring a technician or aide to run the machines is not physical rehab. A licensed physical therapist with advanced training in canine rehab should be on staff in every canine rehab department.

Physical therapists have a unique and specialized skill set that veterinarian-trained rehab therapists do not have. Simply put, physical therapists and veterinarians have completely different educational backgrounds. Physical therapists provide expertise in rehab and manual skills, with a solid understanding of biomechanics, functional anatomy and kinesiology. It's not about one profession being better than the other, it's about realizing that each profession has been trained in different aspects of health care, and we can and should work together side by side to provide comprehensive care of mutual clients.

The Struggles
On a clinical level, it is difficult to hone my skills and brainstorm solutions to unique issues when there are no other qualified practitioners with whom to consult. In human practice, I was always one of a few other clinicians. This enabled all of us to work together and bounce ideas and techniques off each other in order to come up with the best treatment strategy. I don't have the benefit of this collaboration as the only certified rehab professional at Hydropaws.

Another unfortunate struggle is the apparent turf war between the professions of physical therapy and veterinary medicine. Given the obvious track record of success with canine physical therapists rendering canine rehab services, I have yet to understand why some veterinarians resist the development of this practice. I can only assume that some see this as a threat to their practice, that we are somehow taking a piece of the "veterinarian pie." This attitude in veterinarian medicine deeply saddens me.

Currently in the state of California, the Veterinarian Medical Board (VMB) is seeking to add language in their practice act, which would put qualified therapists such as myself under the direct supervision of a veterinarian. This heavy-handed approach is defended by the VMB as a way to protect the consumer (which is indeed their job!). Unfortunately, what this kind of regulation does is limit the consumers' right to choose who they want to treat their pets. To protect this right, the California Association of Animal Physical Therapists (CAAPT) is lobbying against this strict, career-limiting language. As a member of this association, we believe that a veterinarian should be required to complete an examination, and physical rehab could commence only after veterinary medical clearance is received stating that the animal is appropriate for treatment.

The physical therapist is trained and equipped to assess and treat. That training includes post-graduate education at either a Master's level or Doctorate level. To place strict guidelines of direct supervision by a veterinarian on a Masters or Doctorate-level physical therapist with advanced training in canine rehabilitation is incomprehensible. The regulation would deter physical therapists from even going into the field if they ever planned to work in California, as it would relegate them to the position of an aide; both monetary compensation and professional respect would be inadequate to entice therapists to pursue the field at all. Furthermore, the lack of canine rehab research is severely lacking; by restricting the pool of practicing physical therapists, the loss of their expertise will slow the advancement of evidence-based research.

Clearly, as in human physical therapy, regulation is needed to ensure the quality of canine therapists. But these regulations should allow advanced, trained physical therapists to work independently (if desired) and to own their own practices, as long as medical clearance is made for each patient, and communication is maintained with the referring veterinarian throughout the rehab process. This similar approach, already incorporated in veterinary practice acts in Nevada and Colorado (2005 and 2007 respectively), will yield the best results for the patients. To date, there have been no complaints of harm or negligence to animals in rehabilitation provided by a physical therapist in these states or any other. The two professions ought to be allowed to work symbiotically for the benefit of our canine companions.

The Ongoing Pursuit of Excellence

Ideally, I would like to attend more continuing education courses. Being on the west coast of the United States, courses offered are few and far between. I observe surgeries when I can and consistently attend local vet lectures and seminars. I have also learned extensively through the Four Leg Rehab online educational website and participate in a VetRehab listserv online chat group, which connects canine rehab practitioners from all over the world.

And finally, I have spent time in other clinicians' practices. One noteworthy experience was spending a week at the Canine Fitness Centre, working with Laurie Edge-Hughes to hone my manual skills and develop new ones.

The Learnings... and Advice to Others

Looking back, I can see that I suffered from a lack of confidence. It is difficult to make the transition from human to canine rehab, not because of the anatomy, or the biomechanics, or the thought process and analytical skills required to assess a patient and develop an effective treatment program; it was simply difficult to navigate the veterinarian profession as a whole. I came from the human side of therapy where I was welcomed into the medical model of patient care and worked with other professionals as a team. Since veterinarian medicine lacks any allied health professionals, I found it very daunting to enter into the field.

You MUST be passionate about what you do. You must NOT be in it for financial gain. Just adding rehab for the sole reason of increased income potential within an already existing practice is a mistake. Rehab clinics are not running to the bank with profits. This can be a very satisfying career, with professional-level salaries. But a successful clinic takes time and requires highly qualified professionals.

Success can be defined in many ways; my definition is whether I have achieved professional competency that yields excellent clinical outcomes, I am continually growing professionally, I get personal enjoyment practicing my craft, and I am adequately compensated financially to help care for my family. Keep your focus fixed on high quality treatment, and excellent clinical outcomes will match your efforts. Once excellent clinical outcomes are attained, people will talk! Business will come to you when you are good at what you do. Your clients and their pets are your best advertisers—they will let others know how good you are, and your phone will be ringing with referrals!

Laurie Edge-Hughes,

BScPT, MAnimSt (Animal Physio), CAFCI, CCRT
The Canine Fitness Centre Ltd
Calgary, Alberta, Canada
www.CanineFitness.com
Laurie@CanineFitness.com
Phone: 1 403 204-0823

In the beginning

I started in 1992, but quite simply, I have had the good fortune to be in the right place at the right time a number of times! Like many others, when deciding upon a career, I was choosing between Physical Therapy and Veterinary Medicine.

I grew up on a ranch; my father is a cow-vet, and for a long time Vet Medicine was my first choice. I chose PT however, because I didn't want to deal with memorizing drugs, doing surgery, or caring about "innards." I liked muscles, bones, and to a lesser extent, nerves (although I did learn to care about them later!). As fate would have it, I twisted my ankle and suffered an avulsion fracture, which meant a cast and then physiotherapy. The latter matched my interests, and I pursued getting into physio school.

Good fortune meets great timing

Upon graduating from the U of A in 1993, I worked for a short time in a hospital setting, but six months later went into a private practice job with Lesley Kerfoot, MCSP. Lesley was already working part-time with horses, and she would come to work wanting to brainstorm on how one might apply things like "muscle energy techniques" for a dysfunctional sacroiliac joint in a horse by walking it on a hill. There was many a lunch hour spent on our hands and knees trying to figure things out! It was through this employment that I had the good fortune to be around when the first meeting that led to the establishment of The Canadian Horse and Animal Physical Therapists Association (CHAP) was held in Lesley's kitchen in 1994!

I was in on the ground level and took as many courses as were offered by CHAP, which at the time were primarily on horses. In 1996, the position of Secretary for CHAP came up, and I naively asked Lesley whether I would be suited for that job, to which she replied in her distinctive Scottish accent, "I cannot think of anyone better, my dear!" I still laugh at that today, as we all know how difficult it is to find people wanting to volunteer their time to do "grunt-work" for a small association, and I was a PT, both alive and breathing! It was a wonderful happenstance, however, as it provided me with access to international animal physiotherapy associations (and their journals). I was a voracious reader: reading international newsletters, books, texts, magazines. I was also still very young in my PT career and was taking several courses to increase my orthopaedic skills. Learning both aspects at the same time meant that I was always trying to figure out how I could apply one to the other!

Horses, dogs and...pigs
Animal-related education came in fits and spurts. We did anatomy dissections (horse and dog), we had courses on equine behaviour and training; we had courses on equine dentistry as it applies to physio, and we had a vet lecture on common conditions in dogs. I took CHAP courses, I organized CHAP courses, and I even catered CHAP courses! In addition to working on humans, I practiced on anything with four legs (horses, dogs, cats, goats, bulls, pigs...). I officially created my business, Four Leg

Physical Therapy in 1996, and I began by doing house calls. I found it very difficult to charge for my time and my mileage, and hence everyone got a very good deal in those days, until I learned how to be a better businesswoman. Your time, your gas and your overhead needs to be covered!

I had a short stint working out of a veterinary specialist clinic as well, but the concept was ahead of its time, and getting referrals was much more difficult back then. It made far more sense to me and my young family at the time to work from a home office and to set myself "work hours" (people will still come if you tell them that you are only available within certain time frames!). I quite enjoyed this experience. In some cases, I made tea for the owners and other times I would set up a three-hour appointment to treat the dog(s) as well as both owners. It was a nice, easy pace that worked especially well, as my kids were preschool-age—and for how busy I wanted to be at the time. I did direct marketing to vet clinics, had a website created, gave lectures to dog-clubs and had booths at dog shows. (A few impressed breeders and agility-dog owners go a long way to build a clientele!)

It went to the dogs

In 1998, CHAP members were complaining that the courses were primarily on horses, and I was encouraged to create a canine physiotherapy course since I had seemed to have a developing business in canine physiotherapy. At the same time, I was contacted by a US company to teach a canine physical therapy course. I spent months and months researching and writing to create the first ever Introduction to Canine Physical Therapy course that was taught in Canada and the US in 1999. Within a year, I joined forces with Cynthia Webster, PT, and we taught the first few Advanced Canine Physiotherapy courses.

In 2001, I then went to Australia to teach their first Canine Physiotherapy course. I really do think that my teaching is what has reinforced my learning over the years. I was invited to lecture at the 2nd International Symposium on Physical Therapy and Rehabilitation in Veterinary Medicine in 2002, and met several international physio colleagues and veterinarians. It was there that I met Dr. Janet Vandyke, DVM, who later invited me to be a staff lecturer for The Canine Rehab Institute in the USA, which I did between 2003 and 2012.

Teaching

My teaching and lecturing has taken me across Canada, the US and Australia, as well as England, the Netherlands, South Africa, Sweden, and more on the horizon. I have been very fortunate to have met so many wonderful people in this industry from around the world!

My board involvement in CHAP (now the Animal Rehab Division of the Canadian Physiotherapy Association), has been constant since 1996: secretary, president, co-chair, chair, past-chair, chair-elect, and now chair again. I have been tremendously lucky to work with and learn from so many great PTs that have knowingly and unknowingly taught me so much about life, business, politics, teaching, practice, discipline, determination, compassion, dedication, spirit, and more. I am in debt to all of those that I have had the good fortune to work with, learn from and teach.

The Rehab Clinic

I opened a small animal rehab referral centre in 2003 with two business partners, Dr. Amalia Rossi Campos, MZV, MS and Dr. Manuel Campos, MZV, MSc, PhD. Surgeries on their own dog brought us together, and the Canine Fitness Centre Ltd was a co-created vision with these two former veterinarians and me, to provide care to animal athletes and dogs whose own-ers/guardians don't think of them as "just dogs"!

Our secondary purpose and goal has been to push the political envelope: requiring that veterinarians submit a referral for their patients to access our services; open the communications be-tween our association and the Alberta Veterinary Medical Asso-ciation; make animal owners more aware of additional health care options for their pets and be the "ground swelling" that cre-ates change in the veterinary industry. I am also very fortunate to have three other fabulous physiotherapists practice with me: Margaret Kraeling, DPT, CCRT; Jennifer Gordon, BScPT, CAFCI, CCRT; and Donna LaRocque, BScPT, CAFCI, CCRT, CERT, as well as tremendous support staff.

Getting the Masters
In 2004, I learned of the Master of Animal Studies in Animal Physiotherapy degree, offered by the University of Queensland in Australia. It really intrigued me as an avenue to enhance my learning and a way to expand the Canadian and US curricula that I was teaching. I didn't know how I would afford to do the pro-gram, but I just knew that I had to find a way. Thank goodness for MasterCard low interest cash advances! I completed my Mas-ters in 2006, and found the educational process to be very re-warding but entirely time consuming!

All in all, I guess I've just been aware of the opportunities as they presented themselves to me and went with my instincts on pur-suing a direction. Sometimes I felt like I was just being pushed along (whether I liked it or not)—like being in a canoe without paddles—now and then I had to figure out a way to steer, but more often than not I just had to trust that I was floating in the right direction. I certainly didn't plan this direction in life, but I have no doubt that I am doing what I am meant to do.

The Canine Fitness Centre Ltd.
I co-own, operate, and practice out of a stand-alone rehab referral clinic that provides canine rehabilitation/physio services. The Canine Fitness Centre Ltd. is 4000 square feet, with two treatment rooms, underwater treadmill (UWT) room, big exercise area, lunchroom, office, waiting area, bathroom... housed in an industrial bay.

We have four PTs, all part time covering an approximately total of 68 "patient contact" hours (not including lunch hour), and often overlapping in time. One full-time and one part-time receptionist, three rehab assistants covering 43 UWT hours, plus cleaning and minimal reception work (only overlap is four hours on a Monday—one assistant does Administration work then). In addition to, one office manager providing three days times eight or more hours per day, plus off-site work for the clinic as well on the other days.

We will typically see 50 – 65 physio cases per week (seen by the therapist), and 25 – 40 UWT cases per week. The majority of our caseload would be categorized as orthopaedic: 25% postoperative, 25% performance dog, and 25% undiagnosed lameness. The remaining cases would consist of 10% neurologic, and 15% geriatric. It really does vary from week to week!

We bill by time. Therapy sessions and underwater treadmill sessions are separated out and billed individually. Generally, the initial assessment is up to 1.5 hours, and the follow up visits are typically 30 minutes. Underwater treadmill starts at 10-minute sessions, and is categorized (and priced differently) for rehab UWT or fitness/conditioning UWT.

The practice

We practice by veterinary referral for any animal that is late, injured, postoperative, or geriatric. We do see some sporting dogs for minor performance issues or general check-ups periodically throughout a dog's sporting or show career. The Canine Fitness Centre has a strong "word of mouth" support-base.

Rehab starts with an initial assessment by one of the therapist. We each make our own pathofunctional diagnosis and set the treatment plan. Follow-up appointments are either divided into a therapist appointment or an underwater treadmill appointment (or occasionally, a modalities-only appointment) with one of our UWT-assistants. Treatment frequency is dependent upon the condition and tailored to suit the owner's capabilities. If the animal is being treated in the UWT (or with modalities-only), I want to see the animal for a physio check-up every two weeks.

The eventual goal is to be able to discharge the animal from active rehab, but maintain the patient on a "maintenance regime" for check-ups/tune-ups every few months.

Marketing

I think that over 50% of our cases come our way by word-of-mouth or an owner-initiated search for rehab services for their dog. The rest have been told to contact us by their veterinarian. (Either way, a request for a written referral is sent to the veterinarian to obtain consent to treat).

However, I consider all of my correspondence back and forth to the veterinarian as one marketing tool. Beyond that, vets that

refer get a thank you note (with some quirky gift and nutty saying) every month. We have just started a quarterly newsletter,
and all of the local vets will receive a Christmas card. (The top 15
referring clinics will get something yummy as well.)

For direct client marketing, we advertise in sporting/show cata-
logues, and I am currently working on an e-newsletter for our
clients. Each time a new client comes in, they get a "Welcome to
the Family" letter, and when they are discharged they get a
"Thank You Note" (that also asks them to thank their vet for referring them).

Additionally, I love to do cross-marketing promotions with pet
supply stores when possible and talks or seminars for local "dog
folk" are very powerful as well.

Over the years, the advertising strategies that have not worked
have been print ads in magazines (unless in conjunction with an
article written by one of our therapists), and I don't think our
street sign is doing anything for us either (it's going away by the
end of the year)!

Laurie's thoughts on why some businesses fail
I think it comes down to several factors in my opinion. First, it is
likely relevant to realize that the majority (80%) of businesses
fail within their first year of existence! Why? Business experts
profess that it is a failure to plan and lack of business acumen.
Marketing experts can point to failures in marketing campaigns
and the lack of structure and systems. Financial gurus claim that
an insufficient financial buffer and long term financial planning
may be at fault. Any of these factors could be at the root of this
phenomenon.

In addition to the components above, these **could be** contributing to this dilemma:

- Building it too big, too quickly, and simply believing "if you build it, they will come". Then sinking under when the rehab-side of the practice is not paying off the start-up loan as quickly as the underwater treadmill salesperson promised them would happen! This is a new field. The public doesn't exactly know what *animal rehab* is! What can it do? Who will it benefit? Is it right for my animal? Beyond the public, non-rehab veterinarians may have exactly the same questions. The practice of animal rehab has yet to be researched in such way as to be able to state that "rehab for dogs speeds healing, reduces pain, improves customer satisfaction, etc." (That being said, all of the proprietary research on how specific modalities or manual techniques work, were all done on animals!) nevertheless, for animal rehab to grow, we all need to put an effort into educating the public, our co-workers, and the veterinary profession as a whole, on the benefits of animal rehab.

- The quality of animal rehab is not "up to par," and the public and your referral network may begin to lose faith in the practice of rehab and stop coming for therapy or referring patients. The number one rehab skill that is lacking in many rehab facilities is the ability to perform a full physical (manual) evaluation in order to come up with a pathofunctional diagnosis. A traditional medical diagnosis (aka a pathoanatomical diagnosis) is not sufficient to provide physical therapy and rehab services. A simple diagnosis of postoperative TPLO, for example, does little towards coming up with an INDIVIDUALIZED therapy program. How is the animal functioning? What is the integrity of the front limb joints? Are there spinal or pelvis dysfunctions? Are there myofascial trigger points in muscles anywhere in the body? How should complications be addressed? Can they be adequately identified in the first place? Is the person leading the rehab program/leading the rehab department able to conduct a pathofunctional assessment and diagnosis? There is a number of lameness issues that can be caused by structures not typically identified in a typical veterinary exam—rib or sacroiliac joint dysfunctions, muscle strains or tendinopathy lesions. Is the education level and depth of the person running the animal rehab program adequate? Does a vet or PT who is able to make the pathofunctional diagnosis support the technicians who are performing animal rehab sufficient? Are the vets or PTs routinely assessing the animal throughout the rehab process and evaluating the FUNCTION of the animal? Do you need to add a supervising practitioner to your practice, or do you need to enhance your own knowledge?

- The underwater treadmill is not a magic dishwasher and the laser is not a magic wand! They are simply tools, not stand-alone treatments.

- Marketing! And while this technically takes us back to the first point about why businesses fail in general, I think it holds ever more true to this unique area of practice. Your marketing should be relationship building, multiple points of contact, multi-media, and direct response. Am I talking over your head? Then you may need to get training in this field! (I'm working on a program specific to animal rehab currently!)

- Failure to utilize, practice, and niche. If you don't go home and institute a plan to utilize and practice the skills and concepts you learnt, then they will disappear. What is your plan to keep your skills and build your skills? A full rehab facility is likely daunting to many individuals, so in those instances, don't try to serve all rehab. Niche! Perhaps focus on how you can help just the geriatric, osteoarthritic dogs. Perhaps focus on providing just advanced manual diagnostic capabilities and prescribing therapeutic exercises to benefit diagnostically challenging patients. Perhaps focus on the sporting dog clientele. You may need to set aside "rehab days" where your focus on rehab (assessments and treatments) occur on those days only.

Laurie's strengths

I think it boils down to a few different things:

- I like to talk to people and get to know them. I think this is invaluable in establishing a rapport with the clients.

- I have grown up with animals and seem to have an innate sense of "animal body language" translation, which helps me to establish a rapport with the patients.

- My experience and continuing education in "human physiotherapy" has solidified my ability to "know what to do" and treat every case individually.

- My teaching has definitely solidified my knowledge and skills and given me inspiration to continue to develop new techniques or apply different "human theories or techniques."

- I love marketing.

- I guess, I've been gutsy enough to just get out there and "do it"!

- I've had wonderfully supportive people in my life!

In addition, I like to read research papers. That is one thing that I credit my master's degree for teaching me how to do! As well, I like going to the human physio conferences and listening for those golden nuggets of information that I can apply to canine patients.

Laurie's challenges

From a personal perspective, the greatest struggle in practice continues to be how slow political changes and progress are made. Veterinary medicine has no history, practice, or formal education in inter-professional collaboration, and physiotherapists engaged in animal rehab are charting new territory every day!

Also, bear in mind that my practice is comprised of only rehabilitation therapists with a background as physiotherapists. We had a veterinary rehabilitation practitioner with us at the clinic for two years, but she was made to leave our clinic by the veterinary association, because the Canine Fitness Centre is not a veterinary clinic (owned by a veterinarian).

Laurie's advice

As a general statement, I see that most practitioners from the veterinary profession need to strengthen their foundation of rehab knowledge and skill. I think the best way for vets and techs to continue to learn is by collaborating with a physical therapist or learning from physical therapists that can impart the clinical reasoning, foundational rehabilitation sciences, and rationales behind therapy choices and planning as well as refine the manual skills that are fundamental to the practice of animal rehabilitation and physiotherapy.

For physiotherapists, time spent learning animal handling, behaviour and developing a respect for veterinary medicine is a must. Beyond those things, physiotherapists would do well to learn from each other and be inspired by how other PTs/physio are applying their skills and knowledge to animal patients.

I would love to see inter-professional collaboration become a key pillar in animal health care. I am afraid that the veterinary boards/associations will set policies and bylaws based on protectionist attitudes versus open-mindedness, a willingness to learn from and respect other professionals, and a desire to collaborate.

Final thoughts

I see my role moving forward as being a catalyst for political change within the veterinary and physiotherapy professions. I would like to continue my role as a canine physiotherapy/rehabilitation educator and help to guide research in this field of practice.

The need for educational opportunities is why I created both this book and my new educational website www.FourLeg.com.

.

Margaret Kraeling,

DPT, CCRT
The Canine Fitness Centre
Calgary, AB, Canada
Phone; 403-826-9312
Email: margaret@caninefitness.com
Website: www.CanineFitness.com

Margaret's "best laid" plans

My original plan when considering university was veterinary medicine. However, somewhere along the line, I changed my mind and applied to physiotherapy school. I grew up on a farm and was always used to having an assortment of animals around. This translated in later years to involvement in dog sports, especially agility. I took my first canine rehab course primarily because I was interested in identifying and dealing with any potential injuries in my own dogs. I became fascinated by the scope of canine rehab and found it a challenge to apply our research and manual techniques from the human field to our canine patients. It has continued to be a fun challenge every day that I come to work. I just wish I had done this years ago!

Margaret's work today

All rehab clients come to us (The Canine Fitness Centre Ltd) with a veterinary referral. Many times the owner will contact us first and then the clinic will initiate the referral from the vet. Other times it will be a direct referral from the veterinarian. The client will then be booked for an initial assessment of 75 minutes in which an evaluation is conducted, a treatment provided (including a home program), and a treatment plan set up.

We are a stand-alone referral based animal physiotherapy practice. The caseload is primarily orthopaedic (65%), plus geriatric 10%, fitness/performance 15%, neuro 10%, with four rehab therapists and three aides on site. I personally would see 16 – 20 per week. The clinic could see anywhere from 40 – 90 appointments per week between new assessments and follow-ups with rehab therapists. In addition, there would be underwater treadmill appointments. Our charges are based on the amount of time booked for a specific appointment.

The hesitancy of some in the veterinary community to accept the physiotherapists (certified canine rehab therapists) as a valuable member in providing care for their rehab cases can be difficult. I am fortunate to practice in an established rehab clinic with excellent owners who are constantly advocating for improved communication with our referring veterinarians.

I continuously use all my physiotherapy training, most particularly many years of manual therapy, as well as several years in TMJ practice and years of study in craniosacral therapy. All of these techniques are easily and effectively applied to the canine patient. I am continually upgrading my knowledge and techniques with online continuing education as well as journal reading.

The future is bright

As I am nearing the end of my physiotherapy career my focus is on continuing to perfect my treatment skills to benefit my canine clients. This will involve continued learning and interaction with other practitioners. Communication is so essential with the referral veterinarian as well as the client. Clients need to have a clear explanation of the issues as well as the therapist's plan to address them. The owners need to be completely involved in the treatment process. They often have questions after they leave and should feel that they are able to communicate with the clinic/therapist.

I would love to see the time when we are accepted as a valuable member of the team—without hesitation. And even though the educational learning opportunities within the field are definitely lacking, the recent online continuing education (Four Leg Rehab) is filling a huge gap!

My advice for anyone wanting to get involved with rehab would be to have a very **sound** knowledge base (not only in the practice of canine rehab but a general knowledge of the "dog world" in a variety of areas such as sports, breeding, showing, dog breeds). If you are involved in any of these areas—even better. Then good communication skills are important to convey how your expertise can benefit the owners and vets in managing rehab conditions.

Marty Pease,

PT, CCRP
Previously with Canine Rehabilitation and Conditioning Group (CRCG)
Denver, Colorado (previously), & Connecticut (currently)
Contact for CRCG: www.dog-swim.com & 303-762-7946
Personal contact: mcconlogue@msn.com

How did you get started?

As a teenager I had wanted to be a veterinarian. However, I was discouraged from going into the field in the early 1970s by my hometown veterinarian because I was a woman. I had forgotten all about it until I became bored and needed a change of career after 17 years of physical therapy practice. At the time I was working in an outpatient Workman's Compensation clinic, well paid, one patient per hour, and an awesome boss—but bored to death. I recaptured my desire to work with dogs. One of my bosses was treating her veterinarian, who felt that physical therapy should be offered to dogs. My boss put me in touch with him. He and I developed post-operative protocols, and through him I made contact with a specialty clinic that was looking to start a canine rehabilitation practice. That clinic became my main referral source over the next 12 years. At an introduction to canine rehabilitation class I met another veterinarian who got me started at her clinic, and by 2004 I was providing contract rehabilitation services at seven clinics and also working on-call human physical therapy one day a week. My former physical therapy boss had allowed me to gradually cut my hours as I built my canine career. Once I reached 20 hours per week with canines, I made the leap 100% to the dogs (except for the one day a week of human on-call work.)

At the specialty clinic, I met my future business partner. She had a lifetime dream of creating a whole health clinic for dogs. After a year of planning, we opened Canine Rehabilitation and Conditioning Group (CRCG), a freestanding physical therapy clinic for dog rehabilitation. Two years later the Colorado Physical Therapy practice act changed to where it was legal for physical therapists with appropriate training to work with dogs without requiring veterinarians to be on the premises. I stayed with CRCG for seven years until it became time to move back to Connecticut to be closer to my aging parents. At this time, I am working with humans, which I am really enjoying, though talking about canine rehabilitation brings a huge smile to my face.

The information provided below is relevant up to September 2011. I cannot speak to CRCG's status at this present time.

Tell us about the practice

CRCG has three locations. It consists of two freestanding private clinics, and one clinic within a specialty hospital. Two locations have a large pool each for recreational swimming. Each location was a swim-in-place pool and underwater treadmill, laser, electrical stimulation, ultrasound, exercise area and equipment, and acupuncture is provided at two of the locations. Another aspect of CRCG's business was providing consulting business services for canine rehabilitation practices.

For all of CRCG: We utilized two veterinarians and three physical therapists, providing the equivalent of four and a half full-time practitioners, two and a half full time vet technicians, and two full time receptionists. All locations are open six days a week.

One location has one practitioner and is open 40 hours/week, seeing an average of 35 visits/week. The second clinic has one and half practitioners, and is open 52 hours/week, seeing 50-70 visits/week. The third clinic is usually staffed with two practitioners every day, open 56 hours/week, seeing an average 100 visits/week.

Our caseload consists of 5% conditioning (not counting recreational pool use), 40% geriatric, 15% neurologic, and 40% orthopedic. Hydrotherapy is billed as one fee, regardless of the time. All other services are billed in 15-minute increments, consisting of any combination of services. Prepaid packages are offered for all services; five or ten visits can be purchased for a 5% or 10% discount respectively.

The initial visit is 75 minutes and consists of the taking of a history, an evaluation, provision of home program instruction and some form of treatment. Treatment may consist of hydrotherapy, exercise, laser, massage, etc. The follow-up treatments are usually scheduled once or twice a week, and are 30-45 minute in duration. Often hydrotherapy is used in combination with exercise, modalities, or manual therapy.

Referrals and marketing
Often, the client initiates solicitation of rehab services, but a referral to treat is obtained from their vet. The majority (75%) of referrals come from specialty centers, and the rest come from general veterinary practices.

CRCG's marketing strategy was twofold—directly to vets and directly to the public. For the general public, CRCG attended dog events with booths, advertised in publications, held holiday open houses, word of mouth, and hosted "dock diving" events. For vets, advertisements in professional publications, continuing education offerings at their clinics, and client reports. The most successful strategy was the continuing education offerings to clinics. Advertising in local dog publications is hard to track but probably yielded the least bang for the buck. Also CRCG's relationship with the Canine Rehab Institute made more people aware of CRCG's existence. Providing internships for both the University of Tennessee and Canine Rehab Institute students exposed CRCG nationally.

Where have you been successful and where have you struggled?

I think my strengths lie with my love of the work, honesty, integrity, and ability to develop a rapport with vets. I have additional training in energy healing, and dogs are very sensitive to intention of touch and aware of the practitioner's frame of mind. If you are relaxed and centered, the dog will relax. If you are uptight and nervous, the dog will not cooperate. Energy healing education teaches centering and the importance of the quality of touch.

I feel that I struggled with the business side of practice. My business partner handled all the business aspects, but being an owner and manager stressed me out and diminished my enjoyment of the work. I personally am not cut out to be a business owner, and the stress of the bottom line and managing employees wore me down. Though CRCG has been around seven years and continues to be open, it was a nonstop struggle to make ends meet. I feel this was because the overhead (equipment and rent) was so large.

What, in your opinion, has led to failure of other rehab practices?

Too much overhead, non-effective marketing, not enough focus on marketing, to name a few reasons. Locations within a general veterinary hospital sometimes struggle because surrounding veterinarians are hesitant to refer. Any practice that has a rehabilitation practice within their doors needs to make a complete commitment to the success of that practice, including referring clients. Veterinarians often don't realize how time intensive rehabilitation is and that is very difficult to treat more than one dog at a time. This is not how veterinarian clinics are usually run. Often rehabilitation practices are not the money generator veterinarians feel it will be because of the overhead and the time required.

Comment on your continuing education and that within the field in general

Honestly, I'm not very good at this! I don't tend to keep up, but I do attend continuing education events, and enjoyed participating with CRCG's affiliation with the Canine Rehab Institute (CRI).

I do commend CRI for continuously trying to develop courses that meet people's desires and to be willing to add new ones. The international symposium is interesting, but the material presented tends to be too basic; as well, the continuing education classes that meet the skill levels of experienced practitioners in general are hard to find.

Prediction for the future of canine rehab

I do see this as a growing field and who knows what its true potential is. Because it is a cash business, it probably won't reach the level of human physical therapy. As the awareness of the public and veterinary industry grows, the field will grow. As practitioners' interest grows, there will be more and more clinics offering canine rehab. Time will tell if there is enough business to go around.

Any advice?

Start small and within the confines of what you can afford. Grow a little at a time. Freestanding clinics, in my opinion, are more likely to be successful. Have another personal source of income while your canine work grows. And lastly, build a strong relationship with the local veterinarians so that you have a solid basis to grow on and work towards establishing (and maintaining) a good reputation.

Nigel Gumley,

DVM, Diplomate, American College of Veterinary Practitioners (Canine/Feline), CCRT
Cedarview Animal Hospital: www.cedarviewanimalhospital.com
613-825-5001, drgumley@sympatico.ca
Ottawa, ON, Canada

Tell us about yourself, Nigel!

I have membership and affiliations with IVAPM (the Internationalal Veterinary Academy of Pain Management: www.ivapm.org), the AARV (the American Association of Rehab Veterinarians: www.rehabvets.org), the Ontario Veterinary Medical Association, and the Canadian Veterinary Medical Association. I've only been practicing in canine rehab since 2009, but I wish I had started sooner!

How did you get started?

Well, funny you should ask. I can blame it all on my technician, Sarah, who is a constant spark and highly motivated individual. I had been working with her for the four previous years, during which time she had undertaken to develop her training in a number of areas of practice, adding to an increasingly long list of accomplishments. She came to me one day and enthusiastically suggested that she would be interested in learning about rehabilitation, with that look in her eyes that told me that she had her hooks already in her next endeavour. Trouble was that she couldn't take the course without working alongside a therapist, and she wanted me to consider taking the courses with her. At that time, I had a very long-term and dedicated clientele, with a number of geriatric pets among them, and as I considered the proposal, I thought that this would fit very nicely in providing an advanced level of care to this segment of the pet population that we looked after. The rest, as they say, is history. Not only have we succeeded in providing a very beneficial adjunctive therapy to assist with age-related mobility problems, but we very quickly earned a positive reputation among the sports dog community, as well as an increasingly referral practice for area veterinarians.

What does your rehab practice look like?

We operate out of a newly established general practice of 2500 sq. ft. space. We have three exam rooms, a dedicated room for an underwater treadmill, and a couple of other rooms crammed with rehab equipment. Within two years at this facility, we have already determined that we need more space to accommodate the rehabilitation practice, and we are looking for additional space.

Presently, we see approximately one to two new cases per day, and run eight to ten pets daily for treatments four days a week. Our caseload breaks down into 30% surgical orthopaedic, 10% neurologic, 30% fitness or sports injuries (non-surgical), and 30% geriatric or lameness of undetermined origin as the referral. To conduct rehab we utilize one part-time physiotherapist, myself as a vet, and one rehab technician. We often have additional aides to support the rehab practice as well.

Initially, our referrals were from our own client base, or from the sporting-dog community. However, more recently we are getting increasingly higher numbers of patients from other clinics, due to either client requests or direct referrals from other veterinarians. We have a strong relationship with area surgeons but see an increasing number of cases from area general practice vets. The surgeons within the community will recommend us for rehab of their patients with problems surrounding surgical recovery, but not so much for routine care. Many clients find us by a search of their own, and often, there has been a recommendation made by another client. We have many sports-related pets come to us from recommendations made within dog clubs, etc. We have done very little external marketing, relying more on word-of-mouth.

In regards to pricing and continued therapy, we have a referral fee for initial veterinary assessments that are one hour in duration, or a fee to see the PT for a non-vet assessment. We have a fee for 20, 30 and 40-minute treatments, and packages of six and ten treatments, with or without the use of the treadmill. We used to charge by modality but found that it was simpler and more reasonable to charge for the time and use whatever modalities/therapies we needed at a fixed fee. Most clients opt for the packages once the initial assessment is performed, as therapy will take at least four sessions. My technician, Sarah, sets up a therapy program based on my assessment and conducts the treatments. I will conduct periodic rechecks to assess progress and establish new goals, therapeutic suggestions. I leave it up to Sarah to choose the specific therapies that work best for the patient. I will also refer to our PT for advanced manual therapies, IMS [intramuscular stimulation], acupuncture, or for consultation with cases where progress is not advancing as hoped.

What have you done to increase you market share?
We did an initial broadcast mailing to all area vets and included a brochure. We have provided a presentation to clinics that have requested it, although this has been only a small number. We have given talks to area dog groups and have held our own fitness classes (concentrating on core stability) to pet owners.

Overall, advertising has been "soft," relying mostly on word-of-mouth. My concern was that we didn't promote ourselves too aggressively until we were confident in the results. Now, it seems that advertising is unnecessary, as word-of-mouth is so strong.

Why do you think that some animal rehab practices fail and what have you done to avoid this in your practice?

Opening an animal rehab facility or specialty in a market not used to rehab can be a problem. There is a certain period where "training" of local vets is needed to teach the benefits of rehab. A fine line exists between offering a product that is unproven and failing to advertise a service that is mostly successful. It only takes a couple of poor outcomes to turn off referring vets or to negatively affect your reputation. In addition, relying solely on rehab during the growth phase can be risky in a market that is not accustomed to the therapy. Diversifying the income sources can help. And, as with every new business, failure often occurs when one underestimates the risks, overestimates the benefits, and does not look into the long-term goals.

We elected not to promote ourselves too heavily until we were confident that we had a proven service with a history of good results. We worked to fine-tune our skills, learn the equipment, and slowly build a reputation. I was initially concerned about overselling ourselves without having a mature service to offer. Now that we have gotten to a point of confidence and competence in our skills and service, advertising is not overly useful and the word-of-mouth effect of advertising is so strong.

I think that starting off by adding the rehab to a general practice helped, as we were not dependent on one source of income. Additionally, being thorough with lameness or mobility-problem cases has distinguished us from other vets when working up the problem. Rehab has taught me a REALLY GOOD set of exam skills. The biggest strength has been using my technician for treatments, as she offers very dedicated and personalized care, which resonates with the high-end owners who seek out this service.

What about continuing education?

CRI (www.caninerehabinstitute.com)
and Therapaw (www.therapaw.com) offer excellent hands-on courses. For me, my biggest obstacle was getting my head around the science of rehab, as the literature has not been taught in vet school historically, and admittedly, there is a wide variation in quality of evidence, as well as modalities and products offered. There has been a number of things lumped under the rehab banner; each needs to be considered on its own merits. Despite this, there are very sound manual therapies and examination skills that have been taught in the classes, and the instructors are very approachable during and after courses.

What has been you biggest struggle in canine rehab and what advice would you give other practitioners?

Teaching the veterinary community of the unique services of rehab has been a challenge. There is a notion that rehab is primarily a post-surgical benefit for TPLOs, tendon injuries, etc., and while this is true, the majority of our patients fall into other categories. Other clinics have added "rehab services" for post-surgery, but lack the diagnostic skills for subtle lameness issues, or problematic surgical recoveries. Differentiating between the two extremes of rehab is a challenge to a relatively uneducated market. Interestingly, numerous clients are more savvy and experienced, likely due to involvement in the dog-sport community or with their own physiotherapy experiences. Also, the space required for rehab has exceeded what we thought we would need. The vet clinic pays premium rent for location, but the rehab does not need to be in such an expensive location once the diagnosis and treatment plan is established.

I would advise others to spend some time in a rehab practice—there's nothing like seeing cases first hand and practicing your skills. Reach out to the sporting dog community; it's huge and these people are very dedicated dog owners who will talk up your service. Network with others who are offering complementary services such as massage, chiropractic, and acupuncture. Don't try to start a total rehab practice with no other income unless the market is used to what you are offering, as it can be a slow build. Having skilled therapists and assistants is everything. I do not have time to provide the treatments, so I defer to the PT and assistant to do this. I think the technicians are highly valuable and should be considered as more than assistants. I see myself as the diagnostician, and the technician and PT as therapists, with different skill sets.

What do you see as being important to the future of animal rehab and what is your next step?

Integration with pain management is a truly important piece of "good rehab." My vision is to develop ourselves as a Pain Centre, using rehab, acupuncture, pharmacology, and other modalities and to integrate them into a multi-modal service to deal with both acute, and more importantly, chronic pain. We plan to spin the rehab treatments off to a separate and larger facility, as they are outgrowing our space and do not require the expensive rent that the clinic is paying. I have almost completed my certification in pain management, and hope to learn medical acupuncture and IMS in the future.

Robyn Roth,

PT, APT, MPA
Sugarland Ranch, Inc
http://www.sugarlandranch.org
Reno, Nevada
robyn@sugarlandranch.org
(775) 970-5350 telephone
(775) 970-5183 fax

In the beginning

I graduated as a physical therapist in 1971, obtained my MPA in 1979, and obtained Case Manager Certification in 1999. I've had an eclectic career, and physical therapy has been very good to me and me to it. I have practiced in many clinical settings, including pediatrics, home health, acute care, outpatient, wound care, public health and have worked as a clinician as well as having the privilege of being a CEO of organizations, including Visiting Nurse Associations. I also was employed by a top consulting firm and traveled the USA with a variety of consulting projects; I established my own consulting business after the firm I worked with was purchased by one of the "big 8" firms.

In 1998, I started animal physical therapy course work. Clinically, I worked directly with boarded small animal veterinary surgeons, initially Dr. Steve Petersen and since 2003, with Dr. Davyd Pelsue. An opportunity arose to partner with a veterinary surgeon as hospital administrator concurrent with establishing and operating an animal physical therapy department. Those plans were abandoned; however, that planning experience provided insights into the business of veterinary medicine and was likely one of the best educational and preparatory experiences for establishing my private animal physical therapy practice. In 2004, I was one of two physical therapists in Nevada who were invited by the Nevada State Board of Veterinary Medicine to begin working collaboratively to establish a licensing classification for animal physical therapists.

Prior to relocating to Nevada, my husband and I started ground up residential care facilities for developmentally disabled children and adults; however, we both had a passion for animals and knew someday we would be working with animals. I was unaware at the time that this ground up construction experience would be valuable when we developed Sugarland Ranch (our non-profit Mastiff rescue association) in 2001 after re-locating to Nevada. Our business experience and prior consulting experience contributed to developing both Sugarland Ranch and Animal Rehabilitation of Reno/Tahoe. Together, we had already started rescue work with our Mastiffs.

While living in California and after selling our residential care home operations in order to re-locate to our newly acquired land in Nevada, I happened to meet a physical therapy colleague who was working with horses. At that time, at least in California, it was quite difficult to be working with animals unless you were a veterinarian, and honestly, at that time, many of my own colleagues thought the idea of providing physical therapy to animals was absolutely crazy—some thought it was "cute." Insurance was impossible to obtain. Some visionary DVMs began to see the benefit and saw a future for animal physical therapy. At that time, in the late 1990s, David Levine and Daryl Millis at the University of Tennessee were starting to get some articles published and being recognized for their work in animal rehab, as well as Dr. Robert Taylor in Colorado. They were wonderful mentors and provided a great source of information. As well, Lin McGonagle from New York was instrumental in getting a small group of us established as a special interest group within the American Physical Therapy Association.

Fortunately, a colleague in Sonoma County, CA, was receptive to me when I contacted her; she invited me to travel with her as she made ranch calls. She was already working with an equine DVM, who was ahead of his time and "protected" her in her practice in the California environment. There were no regulations at that time and many DVMs felt threatened. However, for the most part in those early years they ignored us because they didn't take us seriously. I was very fortunate that my colleague provided me with a venue for early hands-on experience. Our own DVM was excited about the future of rehab. He practiced both western and eastern veterinary medicine. I started to intern with him, and I kept records on all my hours, somehow knowing that I might need this information in the future. I started taking the courses offered by the APTA, as well as any other courses offered, and in the early years, those courses were offered in Canada. It is at this point that I met the dynamic Laurie Edge-Hughes. As the years progressed, more courses were being offered, and of course, in 1999 the first International Symposium was held in Oregon, which I attended. I have attended all of them, excluding the symposiums offered outside of the USA. I was a presenter in 2002. In the beginning it was a relatively small group of practitioners, and we knew that this new emerging field was going to need to catch up in terms of creating an evidence-based practice. There was lots of discussion of practice models, educational requirements, and there was little agreement, but at least there was agreement that we all wanted to move forward and that some type of education and credentialing was needed. There were, of course, the European models, as animal physical therapy was already well established in countries like the Netherlands and Great Britain, so there were other models to examine—countries that were far ahead of the USA.

The move towards practicing

When I first started, I didn't have any equipment or a practice setting and was also involved in what I termed my "internship" in California, so I relied on home visits or seeing the patient and client initially at the veterinary practice. I also set up a small area of my house to see patients. All of my work was upon the referral and indirect supervision of the DVM. We held routine case conferences, and after practicing as a human physical therapist, documentation was standard; however, collaborating with the DVMs to make it all meaningful to them and ultimately to enhance animal patient care was a learning experience. I also continued to travel with my PT colleague in California as time permitted. (At that time, I was also still working for a home health agency after returning to clinical practice after my time as a consultant, etc.)

Once we relocated to Nevada, our goal was to build our nonprofit, Sugarland Ranch. I was employed as an Administrator of a Rehab Hospital and soon linked up with Dr. Steve Petersen, a boarded small animal surgeon, who was practicing in the Reno/Sparks, NV area. I still didn't have a private practice of my own, so I continued to work at the Vet's clinic as well as home visits. Providing home visits came very naturally as that's what I did in human medicine. By this time I continued to purchase equipment, including a therapeutic ultrasound, laser, electrical stimulation units, mostly portable, proprioceptive equipment, theraband, etc. All the initial equipment was purchased outright without any debt, with exception of the laser. It was the first piece of equipment that I leased, which made business sense at the time. I was also traveling south to the Minden/Gardnerville area on a monthly basis to assist a general veterinary practice with what we termed a monthly "rehab clinic." Those visits were packed, attempting to get as much teaching and patient care done as possible in a short time frame. Veterinarians and technicians were supportive and provided a positive environment for rehab operations. At one time, we even considered starting up a satellite down in that area; however, I got so busy in Reno, it was clear that I had to make some decisions and set priorities. This was a tough call, and by the time I opened my private practice in Reno, time didn't permit to travel south any longer. They continued to refer patients to me even though it took about 60 minutes to get to my private practice.

In 2004, my husband and I planned and constructed our kennel operations, which ultimately became Sugarland Ranch, sitting on 52 acres overlooking the Sierra Nevada Mountains. There were many construction delays and unexpected costs, so the building had to be trimmed down, and there went my rehab clinic—until 2006, when we put an addition on the building. In 2006, I finally got an underwater treadmill, therapeutic pool, a fully equipped private practice clinic. I had an assistant part time, and by 2007 I was seeing on average 8-10 patients per day or average 40 visits/week, some more, some less. I continued to see patients at the veterinary surgical practice and was also involved in doing their post-operative discharges. As my practice continued to grow and as scheduling discharges with a PT became more of a logistical challenge for the surgical practice, this program was abandoned and the surgical practice continued to refer patients to the private practice.

The daily functioning of the practice

I have now semi-retired, allowing me to work full time with our non-profit organization, so I no longer see patients on a regular routine basis. When I had my private practice up and running, I had one "assistant" (not a licensed veterinary technician, as an LVT in Nevada would have required a DVM to supervise them on site). The "assistant" whom I hired was well known in the community; she was very familiar with animals, and in fact, had been a previous rehab client of mine.

As far as charges, I ended up charging by the visit, likely because this is the system that I was the most accustomed:

- An evaluation visit was 60 minutes and a routine visit was 45 minutes, and I also included documentation time.

- The client signed a consent and financial agreement on the initial visit and they understood that if time went over the standard time, then they were charged by 15-minute increments thereafter.

I found that for the most part people did not take advantage of the courtesy extended to them in many cases when they were traveling long distances to get to me, so at times the additional charges were waived. Although I did lose some revenue opportunities, fairness and being reasonable came back to me many times over later in our non-profit; people never forgot what I did for them and their dog.

I guess I'm at peace with my way of doing things, and at the end of the day I can sleep knowing I was always fair. Also, in creating a charge structure, I was aware of what the specialty DVMs were charging for a consult, and in setting my charges, I tried to always charge a little bit less than they did, reinforcing the relationships I had built over the years and to avoid any questions or concerns regarding my charges. So as their charges increased, mine would also increase but always staying slightly under (even though my time with a patient always outweighed the time they spent with a patient). What I tried to avoid is what I term "nickel-diming" people, which I found early on in various careers was distasteful to people, and that although they might tolerate it, they didn't like it.

Referrals and Professionalism
The majority of referrals came from veterinarians, but as the years progressed, more and more consumers would contact me directly, at which time I always would consult with their veterinarians prior to initiating any services. When we developed the licensing regulations in Nevada (2004) for physical therapists, referral patterns were then clarified.

I was also wary about ensuring that the regular veterinarian (RDVM/primary) was comfortable that I would not circumvent him/her and attempt to facilitate patients away from them to the boarded surgeon to whom I was associated, and this association was widely known in the community. Even in some cases where I thought a referral might be appropriate, this discussion remained between the RDVM and me. Although this approach may be perfectly logical, I have directly known PTs who have broken these professional relationships by doing exactly that and circumventing the referring veterinarian and sending the client to one of the specialists, thus jeopardizing their referral base.

I found that although community presentations are important, they did not necessarily translate to increased referrals. Also, similar to human medicine, you had to constantly be reminding the veterinarians the value of physical therapy to keep the referrals coming. One of the challenges of operating a small business with limited staff is that you must manage to treat the current patients you have in addition to ensuring that you have enough referrals coming in to maintain a healthy revenue base. This can be quite challenging for any small business, and you eventually must come to a decision point relevant to how much do you want to grow and what the costs are to that growth.

I also attended veterinary conferences and met people, especially at local gatherings. I participated in rounds and case conferences when asked by a client and/or a veterinarian, ensuring that all timely documentation going out represented physical therapy standards of care, and I utilized each and every evaluative/consult report and note as a teaching opportunity. I addressed the problems, what was done and the outcomes in a concise manner. I also took lots and lots of videos and pictures and shared these with the various veterinarians and, of course, the clients. I have continued this practice when involved in current cases.

Marketing: What works and what doesn't
Although it provided lots of exposure, doing community events and presentations didn't work as far as generating referrals. Newspaper articles about the practice helped to generate referrals in the short term. The newspaper articles also provided the community with information about animal physical therapy and those practicing in the area.

I did some advertising, but the most effective was veterinarian referrals based on producing outcomes on a case-by-case basis. I built a positive collaborative working relationship with various veterinarians by preparing interesting photos, videos and consistently sending their patients' pictures and videos on a regular basis. I received positive feedback by ensuring these were consistently forwarded to them.

Thoughts on why some clinics/practitioners struggle or fail

I believe people misjudge how much effort it takes to start a business (and continue it, especially in the startup phase) and how much capital one must have. We found that it actually requires at least three times what your business plan tells you it requires, especially if you are building bricks and mortar. Also, the entire process of starting a business or program is typically longer than what the business plan originally outlined, so you need to be prepared for this; if one is not prepared in some manner, it can and, in some cases, does lead to failure.

Perhaps another reason rehab departments and/or businesses fail is that they may be struggling with how to effectively communicate the BENEFITS of what they do. An example may be a therapist who is absolutely excellent with manual therapy, in fact, top of their game; however, that may not be meaningful to the client (or at least they don't believe it is) until the end result. So effectively communicating the BENEFITS in functional terms to selective audiences is a critical factor and trickier than what is initially thought. This part of marketing demands time and thought.

Robyn's strengths and challenges

I believe my positive working relationship with our veterinarians, loving what I do, coupled with the ability to produce a product that was value-added for veterinarians and their patients/clients are strengths. Excellent follow through and attention to detail are strengths. It's also important to be on target with an ability to identify the correct clinical problem, and to communicate that problem and what was going to be done about it in an appropriate amount of time. Conversely, the ability to tell the client and the veterinarian when physical therapy wasn't going to be helpful, and management of tough cases, are critical success factors.

In addition, I think another of the greatest challenges was making it work financially as a business owner while focusing on clinical delivery; this is a challenge most small businesses face. Secondly, growing a business and making decisions about human resources, all the things that remain challenging as you are attempting to maintain a clinical practice. There comes that point in time when you either grow, which means hiring employees and managing them (human resources) or stay a one-man show. This is a tough business transition. At the time I finally got my private practice built in 2006, I had already been practicing since the late '90s and I had already practiced in relatively high administrative positions and/or consulting positions in human medicine, where I was responsible for large numbers of employees. I was also responsible for operations, budgets, etc. and I frankly didn't want to do all of this all over again. I was very happy as a one-man show, and when it came time to make that decision all over again, I made a decision to alter my path. I simply had no interest in supervising people any more.

I maintained a limited medical boarding and inpatient rehab program for a while at Sugarland Ranch and continued to provide support to the surgical practice following the transfer of my private practice to them. I'm out of day-to-day rehab operations and busily going forward with our non-profit mission. For practitioners who make a decision to practice under the supervision of another business owner, the challenges remain ensuring clinical competency, assessment, treatment, outcomes, research, patient and client relations, case management and being an effective team member.

Robyn looks back

I'm very busy with our non-profit and Sugarland operations; however, I regret not pursuing a Doctorate in Physical Therapy—it was a professional goal that I did not meet, at least not yet.

As far as certification, I believe I had already prepared myself with the education I had accrued and a successful private practice, so I did not pursue certification. Further, to practice in Nevada, we had already passed regulations in 2004 based on educational and clinical requirements that were established in addition to continuing education, so certification was not a requirement in order to obtain a license to practice "animal physical therapy." It is, however, an option towards licensure in Nevada. I was well on my way to treating patients full-time by the time the certification courses were organized, but I continue to recommend them to newcomers.

The certification programs make it far easier offering a basic foundation in an organized manner, under one roof, so to speak. If I were continuing full-time in animal PT, I would pursue a DPT and likely take advantage of many of the courses being offered by the various educational programs.

Future of animal physical therapy

I see dual credentialing as one alternative, specifically, DPT/DVM. Another alternative is establishing a master's level program, as I believe other countries have done, available for both PTs and DVMs.

More research and publications need to be forthcoming to validate what we are doing. We are such a relatively new field and have accomplished much, but we have a long way to go. I see more and more DVMs owning the field and establishing rehab practices. Physical therapists must continue demonstrating their value through evidenced based so that we continue to sit at the table. The value of a team similar to the way a human comprehensive rehab program operates is paramount. The ability to effectively communicate this concept and its benefits is perhaps easier said than done.

As our profession continues to move forward, I have given some thought to all the issues that the APTA has faced relevant to POPTS (physician owed physical therapy) and how these issues might be relevant to veterinarian owned practices that employ physical therapists, and how these issues might shape the various future formats for business and professional relationships.

Robyn's advice for newcomers
I would strongly advise anyone planning to construct a clinic to ensure whatever your business plan tells you need in terms of funding, that you triple that number. Many businesses fail because they are underfunded and construction is a difficult game—it seems it always takes more resources than what you planned.

This comment is confirmed by many of the veterinarians I'm associated with who have stated exactly the same thing when building their clinics. The underfunding puts you in a very undesirable position right out the gate. You cannot go back, you must go forward, and you end up with debt that you didn't plan and then you have to run hard to try to make up this deficit. A good and realistic business plan is critical, particularly when it pertains to construction. Always triple the expenses and time that is required, and you should be okay.

We had experience constructing ground up our residential care business in California and also our current Sugarland Ranch, as well as the addition for the animal physical therapy clinic, and we did the latter right before the bottom fell out of the economy. So what I would have done differently is adjusted our business plan accordingly. Of course, no one ever anticipated the tremendous economic failure so many businesses underwent. Mine did not; I simply made a decision to transition it to a veterinary surgeon so that I could go a different direction. As far as those practitioners that do not want to construct a clinic nor own a business, there is a demand right now for qualified practitioners, and I would highly recommend getting associated with a specialist— or if you can, a large referral center—because I think the knowledge that you gain in that setting is so valuable and simply isn't offered in other settings.

Finally, having a solid, realistic and accurate business plan with short and long-term goals. Short-term goals are becoming more and more important due to the uncertainty of economic times, making long-term plans challenging and somewhat unpredictable. For clinicians entering the field, whether business owners or those who elect to work in an alternative business structure with a veterinarian, it may be prudent to at least think about business relationships and what that means for the future. Further, making decisions around what practice/educational models you want to pursue and pursue them. I encourage new physical therapists to look at the certification programs because they do provide a foundation concurrent with pursuing a DPT.

What needs to change?

I see the field becoming more polarized by discipline. Rehabilitation has always been equated to a team approach and always will be reliant on team for success. I'm quite delighted with the way things are progressing but hope that physical therapists continue to be involved with the process and the team. It has been reported to me that the current available certification courses have more and more veterinary technicians and veterinarians enrolled than physical therapists. If this is true, this is a marked change from years ago.

Robyn's final thoughts

Continue growing through education, research and clinical practice by discipline and by team. Learn from others who have gone through the same process so that their errors can be avoided and growth expedited and enhanced. I appreciate all the support and assistance that was graciously provided me by other physical therapists, veterinary technicians and veterinarian colleagues, all of whom furthered my education, knowledge, and continued curiosity. I also want to acknowledge Dr. Robin Downing in Colorado, who has inspired me to pursue my interests in pain management and end-of-life care.

Sarah Sandford (Dalton)

MSc Veterinary Physiotherapy; BSc Hons Physiotherapy
Physio-Vision; www.physio-vision.co.uk;
Phone: 07795 272286
Email: physio-vision@hotmail.co.uk
Essex, UK

How it all started:

I started practicing canine physiotherapy in 2007, working for a few different ACPAT members covering caseloads. I then worked on promotion at four local vet practices/hydro centres to create my own caseload.

Sarah's Working Schedule:

Today, I work with one other physiotherapist at the clinic, seeing about 45-50 patients a week, including equine and canine home visits. The practice sees approximately 60% Ortho, 30% Conditioning, and 10% Neuro. Billing is simply done by time, with either a "new patient" or "follow-up."

Continuing the Practice:

Getting referrals from vet practices is a great way to maintain business, and we do get word-of-mouth recommendations as well, via the website. Being professional and showing skills that can help the clients of the vet practice is one of my strengths. However, the lack of self-promotion and recognition within the practice can be damaging; you need to devote time and persistence with some practices to get the recognition and involvement in appropriate cases. I like to keep current through human CPD and ACPAT courses, as well as journal reading. Generally, the educational learning opportunities within the field are good—seminars and subscription to the Journal of Small Animal Practice and the ACPAT journal.

One of the biggest struggles is managing caseloads, trying to please the client, and also with the travel and losing time and money.

Sarah's Views on the Future:
Going forward I would love to have my own treatment room and to be able to practice acupuncture. However, I will also continue to work using human physiotherapy skills from hand therapy, splinting using thermoplastics, and neoprene for the neuro/ortho cases.

I LOVE doing my job, and the opportunities available are ongoing. If you want to grow your business my advice would be to spend time with other practitioners, be professional and keep up-to-date with the skills and developments available to you.

Shannon Budiselic,

HBSc (Hons. Biology), DVM, CVA, CERT, CCRT
Equilibrium Veterinary Rehabilitation & Consulting Ltd.
Okotoks, AB, Canada
www. equilibriumvrc. com

What's your "story," Shannon?

I tell people that I entered the world of rehabilitation in a very round-a-bout manner, and an interesting unknown fact is that I applied to University of Manitoba's Physical Therapy program after graduating with a Biology degree from Lakehead University in 1998. My mother suffered numerous complications related to multiple head injuries during my childhood. The dedicated PTs and neurologists who assisted with my mother's lengthy recovery inspired me, and I was intrigued by the concept of "neuro-plasticity."

I did not have all the requirements for admission to the program at U of M, but I was preparing a grand move to Alberta from Ontario with my husband as he took his first job as a newly graduated Civil Engineer. My attention then turned to applying to the Western College of Veterinary Medicine in Saskatoon, and after one unsuccessful application, I later graduated in 2005 with my DVM. My CERT (Certified Equine Rehabilitation Therapist, Animal Rehabilitation Institute) training was sparked in 2006 when a client returned to me with a stallion that developed compensatory issues, ultimately culminating in a second surgery, and I had started the process of asking myself, "why is this happening?" My training as a CVA (Certified Veterinary Acupuncturist, IVAS) began in 2008, and I was amazed by the concept of medical (Western) acupuncture and biomechanics. During this training, a long line of clients and friends were approaching me with canine clients, and I began incorporating rehabilitative techniques (self-learning canine applications primarily with therapeutic exercise and basic manual technique) with acupuncture and TCVM management in many cases. In 2008, I started Equilibrium, an outpatient, referral-based rehabilitation and integrative care practice, and established a dedicated list of equine and canine patients ranging from ageing, arthritic "couch potatoes" to performance athletes.

I first learned about Laurie Edge-Hughes years ago, when I began my immersion in the world of rehabilitation, and physiotherapy colleagues kept encouraging me to contact her. In June 2010, after one phone call, and one coffee, Laurie and I had agreed that it might be an idea if we joined forces and attempted collaborative practice at her clinic, The Canine Fitness Centre. The caseload and variety of cases at the facility, and the quality of clients elevated my practice to an entirely new level, and it gave me an amazing foundation for qualifying as a graduate CCRT through Canine Rehab Institute's program in 2011. Unfortunately, we were unable to maintain the working relationship due to regulatory issues, and I returned to solo practice in July 2012. It was a privilege working with Laurie and the other therapists at the clinic, and the fresh perspective contributed greatly to my ability as a rehabilitation veterinarian.

Shannon's workweek

I see upwards of about 20 cases per week with my ambulatory practice. My practice breakdown is about 40% orthopedic, 30% geriatric, 20% sports/fitness conditioning, and 10% neurological (with some overlap in cases, of course).

Equilibrium is an ambulatory practice, and the majority of my work is canine, thus, I visit these patients in their homes, which has the advantage of overseeing activities of daily living, particularly. My work also involves a smaller equine load, and the casework takes me to stables in my local area and throughout the province (on special consult request only—primarily for second or third opinions).

Where do your referrals come from?

The majority of my referrals are directly from veterinary referral centers and from general practicing veterinarians in the Calgary area. The specialist referrals are primarily neurological and orthopedic, while primary care DVMs will refer for a "second or third opinion" on a puzzling case or directly refer for specific conditions. Often, satisfied, loyal clients will recommend my services to their friends and family. Clients will often procure my services for other members of their existing or new dog family, and it is not uncommon to treat numerous generations of dog family members within one household.

How do you manage your caseload?

A referral is obtained from the referring veterinarian to provide rehabilitation therapy and/or provide a second or third opinion on a case. Medical clearance is sought mostly for clients requesting evaluation of a non-lame or non-injured dog from a sport medicine and performance perspective. After a detailed initial assessment of all history and information available, a plan is implemented for continued care and communicated with the referring veterinarian (including specialist) and client. This plan for continued care also considers current medical issues, including co-morbidities, which may impact the patient's rehabilitation. The plan may also involve or suggest further diagnostics or a specialist referral (typically surgical or neurological) for follow-up.

Depending on the case, when a patient is in rehab, they may attend therapy sessions more frequently in the early stages. This allows me to establish a rehabilitation program and guide success towards desired outcomes. Once the primary goals are achieved, the sessions may be sufficiently spaced to a maintenance level, or the patient may be fully discharged. Progress notes are sent back to the referring veterinarian, updating them on the patient's progress throughout the rehab process, and communication regarding specific concerns (i. e. ancillary pain management, or concerns regarding healing or owner compliance), as needed. I also aid the client-general practitioner relationship by reminding the client of co-morbidity monitoring, including regular blood work monitoring in cases of long-term administration of pain or other medications.

Services are basically charged on a per time basis with a foundation rate in mind (with incremental increases on a biannual basis typically). Extra costs apply to assistive devices and for materials and supplies if applicable to the case. The client is typically advised of the approximate charge per visit and the expected number of treatments in the case of a specific related injury (i. e. non-complicated post- surgical TPLO cases tend to be more "routine," and I have a better idea of the expected rehabilitation for these dogs). In typical maintenance-type geriatric cases, I aim to determine an appropriate regular maintenance interval for the animal, from which the client can determine long-term care costs.

Advertising strategies (The good and the bad)
Direct Communication with the Referring Vet—I found that the best form of marketing has been directly communicating

with veterinarians on cases, and specifically providing them with some vital, "point of sale" pieces of information. For example, after the referral, a detailed case report is sent back (by the following day), with considerations for the patient's care by the regular DVM. I include my functional assessment findings and recommendations (including all options) and the rehabilitation goals (and specific outcome measures that I will be monitoring). Clear, direct communication has multifaceted advantages.

Firstly, an open dialogue with your colleagues facilitates ideal patient care. By limiting my practice to rehabilitation, the referring (non-specialist) veterinarian is reassured that I am not going to "steal" their client, but rather I will be working with them as a team member to provide the patient with the best care possible. These practitioners also find reassurance that the patient's overall health needs are considered in my rehabilitation plan, since I often remind clients to visit their regular or specialist vets for monitoring, follow up, blood work, of various existing or suspected "new" co-morbidities as required. Surgeons, in particular, feel reassured that I am not stressing the surgical site with my descriptions of therapy and recommendations and understand that I am also working towards the same goal and protecting their interests. Secondly, from the perspective of the client, good communication reassures that their animal's health care team members are working together in the best interests of their animal, while considering the client's philosophy and financial concerns. Clients really want to do what is best for their animals, and expect us (rehab professionals) to "quarterback" on their behalf. I think this a very important point to make. At the end of the day, we are doing what is best for that patient, and we should aim to work and play well with one another to facilitate this.

Website (and your Online "Track" Record)—A well designed, "clean" and informative website that outlines your philosophy and what you do, including your qualifications and services, goes a long way these days. Many clients will "Google" their prospective health care providers before their first appointment, and they are not embarrassed to let you know this when speaking with you. Living the part of adopting a healthy lifestyle (I've taken up running and cycling for example) also plays an important role in "talking the talk and walking the walk" with your clients.

Rewarding Your Clients—Clients reward me for a job well done when they recommend me to their friends, so I reward my clients with coffee gift cards as a means of saying "Thank You." I also want to start a birthday program for my patients, but haven't gotten around to that yet.

The Bad—I found that the following marketing tactics have *not* worked:

1. Yellow pages ads—Your paper ads need to be in a place where specialty people will look for you (i. e. dog show flyers, or breed review magazines, or specific sport publications);

2. Writing for local magazines in the hopes of passing information on to the general public, who have a general understanding of pet health. I found that my expertise was lost on the individual editors who wanted me to write for them, and the general public, who were not as concerned with access to "specialist" knowledge.

What are YOUR strengths?

I guess I have enough experience and passion for my work to make me a rather opinionated, but very altruistic and pragmatic practitioner (I'm a "straight-shooter," I want to "play fair," do what is best for my clients and patients, and help advance the profession collaboratively). On the lighter side, I am a terribly authentic and nerdy individual with the ability to visualize abstractly and problem-solve. I also have a creative and biomechanical brain, thanks to my father (a fabricator), although I have yet to rival Laurie's quadriceps contracture rig-ups! I think of all of my patients as my "kids" (my clients must think I have an enormous brood of fur children, based on my conversations with them during appointments). I am also very respectful and diligent as a professional, which aids communication and diplomacy. I am also a community mentor to a veterinary student at the University of Calgary, and I am striving to develop my mentorship and leadership skills, which helps with inter-professional development in the community.

What have YOU found most challenging in practice?
I think the biggest challenge I have faced is that my practice philosophy is considered "ahead of its time," so-to-speak, from a veterinary perspective. Veterinary medicine, although historically an old profession, has taken some time to advance relative to human medicine, and the explosion of new veterinary specialties is a relatively recent phenomenon, primarily driven by the needs and expectations of society. For the most part, the current regulatory foundation, at least in this province, is not yet set in place to allow for truly collaborative practice between veterinarians and allied health professionals. Understandably, time and careful consideration are required to ensure that the best interests of all professional parties are considered when forming this framework.

Much of my professional career, by default, has been vouching for the physical therapists that have helped to build this field,

and explaining to veterinarians that PTs are allied-health professionals with a real sense of liability and professionalism, and that
rehabilitation is a well-established field in human medicine. This
not only validates what I do as a rehabilitation professional, it
additionally describes that what I provide is more than a "complimentary modality," and is a supportive therapy delivered in
an entirely new way, which is not inferior to what I did when I
worked in a conventional referral practice.

The second challenge I faced is that I had to get past the concept
of looking at only the patho-anatomical lesion, and the reliance
on that "x-ray," and begin to trust my hands more as my caseload
and experience increased. I like to tell people that if I lost all my
rehab equipment, I would get by with my hands and my brain
(the most valuable and sought after tools I own). These tools
(your hands and brain) give your clients the most useful information, and this is what they are ultimately paying for when they
visit you.

Why do you think that some rehab clinics fail?
I think some rehabilitation facilities and departments fail because there may be an expectation that, "if we build it (the rehabilitation centre), they will come." Practitioners are often ro-
manced by the concept of rehabilitation and excited about re-
vealing a new building and their "toys" rather than selling the
process of rehabilitation, which is in reality a very sobering process. Many veterinary clinics are primary care facilities, and they
attempt to run the rehabilitation side of their practice like a regular clinic. Other primary care clinics may see those practices as
a potential threat; if they send a client there for rehabilitation,
they then cross their fingers that the client's loyalty to their own
practice remains, and that they will return to their practice. Clinics with rehabilitation-added practices may also attempt to run

this side of the practice like a regular clinic: charging per modality (in the veterinary way of making a piece of equipment pay for itself), scheduling shorter appointments, or charging either too much or inadequately (in some cases) for the services. Sometimes, veterinarians simply want to turn the rehab department over to a technician, thinking along the lines that the "modality" is the rehabilitation (rather than providing a full functional assessment each time). This can often lead to failure of case management. Additionally, the clinic may lack a full-time dedicated rehabilitation practitioner who sees a large number of cases on a regular basis in order to build that particular practitioner's rehabilitative clinical reasoning capacity. Problem-solving rehabilitation algorithms are almost entirely different to conventional veterinary reasoning. This fact reinforces the need for regular collaboration between PTs and DVMs in day-to-day rehabilitation practice. PTs and DVMs each put a different, and complimentary, spin on their work, and it is wonderful to be able to pick one another's brains at lunch or between appointments about that "one case."

Another point I am going to reiterate is the concept of rehabilitation as a "modality" based field rather than a "process." Veterinarians in particular are often targets of many modality marketing companies (not that I am picking on companies for promoting their products), and the belief that the rehabilitation modality is the cure-all is prevalent in veterinary medicine. Case-in-point is the fact that many companies are marketing to general practicing veterinarians at trade-shows and conferences, as opposed to marketing and selling to DVMs or PTs with special training in the use of these modalities. We (the trained professionals) recognize that some modalities can be harmful and have contraindications in some cases, of which regular DVMs may be unaware. Plus, veterinarians are often used to charging more for a service rather than for their time or specific expertise, which then exacerbates the modality-based style of practice. The art of rehab practice is not the chosen modality, but the ability to construct a comprehensive treatment plan around a case to ensure a positive outcome. The foundation of success in any rehabilitation program is the functional assessment, and the ability to perform it well, to choose a treatment regime, or to refer for further diagnostics or other interventions, as necessary. A veterinary diagnosis is sometimes not available in many referred rehabilitation cases, and often cases arrive in the therapist's hands with "open" diagnoses. Thus, the rehabilitation practitioner really becomes the patient's "quarterback," and to be a "quarterback" one must certainly define the situation for the patient, and respect, support, and educate other members of the health care team.

Talk about further education, please!
I make a point of attending the IAVRPT Symposium (depending upon the location) and have access to other forums for discussing cases (IVAPM & AARV). I am planning on attending additional CRI CE courses as well. I am also furthering my education in the field of human sport medicine because of my own interest in athletics (topics of athletic conditioning and endurance sports are my passion) and the comparative information that I can transfer back to my canine sport and rehabilitation patients.

I just want to clarify that I have significant experience in this field from all angles (and have been consulted for my opinions), and the opinions expressed in my comments are my own, without directive, although I have many collaborative associations with PTs. The current certification programs (and I can predominately speak for the Canine Rehab Institute, since this was the program I took) certainly provide an excellent foundation for practitioners. I also feel as though the advanced CE options provided are also relevant and valuable.

Education beyond basic certification should involve some board certification or a master's degree of some type, and although I believe these are reasonable options, I am (I guess, altruistically) concerned that continued growth of the profession as a whole will be optimal with continued collaborative inputs from working physical therapists and collaborative academic departments. I am concerned that the gap between physical therapists and veterinarians is widening in the field of animal rehab: skewed class ratios between DVMs and PTs in certification classes; the disappearance of advanced certification or master's level programs for PTs; basic issues regarding legislation, policy, and by-laws; the formation of specific groups and associations that do not include both groups (although some good examples of inclusive groups exist) that fails to support the vested interests of the animal PTs (current and future). Ultimately, rehabilitation is evidence-based at its roots and is not static with respects to requiring inputs from both DVMs and PTs for future growth and advancement of the field. If the premise is that the field of rehabilitation is collaborative and was founded on the backs of PTs, we fail as a whole field, and risk stagnating, and practicing/educating new generations of rehabilitation therapists in a dogmatic fashion if we continue to exclude PTs from the profession (advertently or inadvertently), because the current legislation and structure is unsupportive. If the legislation and structure is still unsupportive, then we need to balance the playing field. I'll get off my soapbox now!

Do you have advice for new animal rehab practitioners?
My typical advice is to do a SWOT (Strengths, Weaknesses, Opportunities and Threats) analysis (thanks, Laurie!), and deter-

mine the basics from that on a business level. On a philosophical level, I tell people to imagine what their ideal day, ideal patient, and ideal client looks like, and to focus on that. I believe in the law of attraction.

The future of animal rehab

I love the concept of ONE-medicine and love how it has become a sexy catch line for academic institutions, but I would really love to see rehabilitation taught as a ONE-medicine topic in veterinary and physical therapy faculties. In particular, explanation of the concept of the functional diagnosis and its application in practice. Some of the best innovations and eureka moments in science and medicine have arisen from collaborative practice—the real art is making it work politically in the "real world" of clinical practice.

Final words

Being a rehabilitation practitioner has proverbially and literally brought me to my knees as a veterinarian in the sense that it has humbled me tremendously, and I now do all of my exams at floor level! The ability to perform a thorough functional assessment is the key to helping my patients, and if I lost all my bells, whistles and toys as a rehabilitation practitioner, I would do more than survive, I could thrive—with my hands as my best tools! Lastly, I want to take just one line to thank all my PT and DVM mentors for believing in me and for pioneering a wagon trail for myself and other homesteaders to follow.

Sonya Nightingale,

MCSP, Grad Dip Phys, ACPAT Cat A, ACE
(Accredited Clinical Educator) Chair of ACPAT 2009 - 2013
Highworth Physiotherapy Clinic,
Highworth, Wiltshire, UK
www.highworth-physio.co.uk

How it all started

I started practicing veterinary physiotherapy in 1988. ACPAT was only formed in 1985 (the year I qualified as a human physio), so animal physio in the UK was very much in its infancy. At that time the human physio course itself was only a diploma, and a vague upgrade route to treat animals was forming, involving shadowing vets and attending a couple of courses over two years. Nothing like the present! From there I started treating animals belonging to friends and relations and going out talking to vets, riding clubs and local pony clubs.

The business

Dogs come to a ground floor room in our clinic (which is a grade two listed building on a small town high street in the UK) as outpatients. We have wooden floors for ease of cleaning but a big non-slip mat on which to assess the animals. Gait assessments are done in the clinic garden or (much to the amusement of the locals) down the sidewalk on the high street.

I travel to see horses in their own yards, though never more than 45 minutes away from base. Some horses with owners who can't carry out the rehab will come to a livery yard close to me, where I have an assistant who does all the day-to-day rehab from instructions she is given; she is an excellent horsewoman and never carries out the therapies if she notices a problem. However, it is the owner that carries out most "rehab" by following therapist instructions.

I normally see two or three dogs, about 20 to 25 horses and 20 to 25 people per week. I work three days a week clinically and spend the last two days either lecturing or attending to ACPAT business, or this year (2012), Olympics administration and organisation.

This is a private practice where all but one of the other physios only treat humans. There are eight of us altogether, and we mainly see musculoskeletal and orthopaedic problems from all age groups. It's a 50/50 split of pet and competition dogs, mainly agility and flyball. Horses are a big mix of riding club to elite eventers, with a few polo ponies in between.

Spreading the news

Word-of-mouth is invaluable and your best tool. People will always ask their friends/trainers/relatives before they go looking in a directory or online. I keep directory entries mainly for people who have lost my contact details and need to know where to find me.

A website with good photos and explanations also helps convince some people who want to "check up on you" before entrusting you with their best friend. Otherwise, talks to clubs, organizations (both professional and general public) works best for me. Surprisingly, talking to riding club members doesn't just bring horse clients; it brings people and dogs, too! My referrals now mainly come from local vets and word-of-mouth.

Sonya's strengths

Being an accredited clinical educator has helped me understand different learning styles, and therefore, helped me vary the way I explain things to owners. Being always approachable and trying to educate owners as much as treating the patient is vital—I use good explanations and a relaxed atmosphere.

ACPAT is a wonderful organization, but I would say that, wouldn't I?
Seriously though, I think we are very lucky in the UK—a relatively small country with a relatively large number of animal physios and a professional organization in the form of the Chartered society that supports us. I glean a lot of knowledge from experience, from other physios and from the vet conferences, etc. Plus, a lot of research!

Sonya's had some challenges

When I started there was very little vet-physio going on and a lot of "bone-setters" floating about. There are still a lot of "cowboys,"' but at least the professionals are beginning to gain recognition and legitimacy.

I think we are constantly battling because we are at a knowledge cliff. What I mean is that it's such a young profession that no one yet knows the answers and research is lagging way behind. A lot of what we do (whether we like it or not) can be a very educated guess.

The profession has changed hugely since I came in and it needs to continue to do so. Professional acceptance by a skeptical veterinary profession is still a big problem; however, it's a very exciting adventure, as we are at the forefront of developments.

Sonya's advice for newcomers

Go on a business course and be realistic. Don't grow too fast in an uncertain market, having large loans you cannot service. Be a people person—owners pay the bills, they have to like and trust you and never feel that they're being ripped off. Never be arrogant or unapproachable!

Be involved with your peers, go to regional group meetings, work with and on the committees—you will get more out of it than you could possibly imagine and get opportunities to go places you can only dream of; your self-confidence will soar!

Once you're established, take students, as they force you to keep thinking and keep dissecting your practice, making you keep up-to-date. Work hard and communicate, nothing comes to you just because you wait; you have to make it happen. If you work hard you can make anything happen!

Sonya's dream

If I won the lottery, I would obtain a one-furlong horse walker with variable speed up to canter to enable more controlled equine rehab for the more nervy ones! Otherwise, I want to be more involved in teaching and practical help for business start-ups.

I would also love to see proper and full recognition and regulation of the profession involving protection of title to stop the "cowboys." I believe we will see people training directly as animal physios, bypassing the human qualification, but this must be via an in-depth, proper, full-length bachelor's or master's degree of at least three years duration, and not via weekend courses. Hopefully, that will come with full professional autonomy and a more workable partnership with the rest of the team.

Final thoughts

Go talk to the vets and other members of the team—they don't bite, and once you get to know them you will realize that they don't know it all and are sometimes just as mystified by a case. Use your professional group and networks; they are invaluable (and also rarely bite)!

Susan Calverley,

DVM, CCRT
Mission Vet Hospital & Orthopets Canada
Mission, BC, Canada
www.missvet.ca & www.orthopets.ca
doctor@missvet.ca & doctor@orthopets.ca
Phone: 604-826-8456

What brought you to where you are today?

My girlfriend invited me along to Arnhem, Holland for the Fourth International Symposium on Physiotherapy in Animals (October 2006), and I got HOOKED! I met Laurie Edge-Hughes, Jan van Dyke, and Bart Menten and came home and signed up for the CRI [Canine Rehab Institute] courses. I spent two summers in Colorado and I was certified in 2009. I also found a human physical therapist (PT) close to home that was in the dog world and also associated with Laurie Edge-Hughes, and we have been collaborating ever since.

I continued my training and took CRI's first course offered in Veterinary Orthotics and Prosthetics, and I met Martin and Amy Kaufman. I was fortunate to get to spend time at their rehab practice with Patsy Mich, and I found my rehab niche in 2011. I have been the Canadian distributor for Orthopets for almost two years now, and I am so excited to be part of this exciting new field within the veterinary rehab profession.

What does your rehab practice "look like"?

I provide rehab within my general veterinary practice and tend to see about three to five rehab cases a week. Our caseload would be about 80% orthopaedic, 10% neurologic, and 10% geriatric. Our team consists of one part time vet, a PT every other week, and a part time assistant. We bill by time—more for the first evaluation and then flat rate for 30-minute therapy sessions.

I get referrals from across the country for orthotics and prosthetics; many of my patients work with rehab practitioners and their regular veterinarians across the country. Local clients are either referred or find us through our internet marketing. Once they are "in," they usually spread their visit between the PT and myself and will initially visit weekly and then go on a maintenance schedule. Sixty percent of our rehab cases are clients of the clinic, 20% are referred by their primary care DVM, and 20% come from veterinary referral centres.

What marketing / advertising strategies do you suggest (or not)?
We advertise via the internet primarily. We find Facebook and veterinary trade shows to be useful. What hasn't worked are client-oriented trade shows and an open house at the clinic!

Can you talk about your thoughts on why some rehab facilities fail and what YOUR strengths have been to overcome this?
I think some facilities start off with far too much overhead (over extend to start), and there is not enough education and "buy in" from primary veterinarians and the economy. I think I have succeeded by finding a niche that fits me and by starting small.

What about continuing education and opportunities for this in the field?

I think that the rehab profession as a whole is very supportive and helpful. I have been able to spend quality time with many private practitioners, and they have been very forthcoming with how they do things and what works for them. There are some really good continuing education courses and conferences out there. (CRI, Laurie Edge-Hughes' website, rehab list-serve, acupuncture with the BVAS, and I am looking forward to MAV at CSU (Medical Acupuncture for Veterinarians at Colorado State University) and trigger points with Dr. Wall. If I weren't reluctant to fly to New Jersey, I would definitely hit the STAAR conference, and I LOVE the CRI courses in Colorado.) Unfortunately, one of my biggest struggles is getting away from practice to attend CE courses and getting enough patients to practice on!

I think to nurture our profession we need to continue what we are doing by mentoring each other and providing supportive environments, like the list-serve, and then start providing more support and education for the primary veterinarians about how we can help their patients and their practices.

What are your goals and next steps in the future?

The next step is to further my acupuncture training with some trigger point and the MAV course at CSU. Acupuncture is an integral part of my rehab practice now. I also want to get the word out about veterinary orthotics and prosthetics to the veterinary profession in general and KEEP PRACTICING!

Thoughts on the future of animal rehab?

I would like to see rehab as a more well-known and accepted modality by the general veterinary profession. I would also like the veterinary profession to be more open to inter-professional collaboration. I would not be able to provide the care that I do without the support of the human physiotherapy field and the human prosthetic field. I have learned so much from them!

And lastly, do you have any words of advice?

Start small, study lots, and find a good mentor!

Tammy Culpepper Wolfe,

DPT, PT, CCRP, GCFP
(GCFP is Guild Certified Feldenkrais Practitioner)
The K9 Body Shop, PC
Arvada, Colorado
www.thek9bodyshop.com
twolfe@thek9bodyshop.com
Phone: 720-447-7268

Tammy's up and down beginnings..."it will pay off"
It all started in 2002. I had a private human practice at the time when I received a CE brochure from Northeast Seminars about a canine course offered in Denver. I immediately considered a change, but wanted more information. I called Marty Pease and Carrie Adamson (now Adrian) to ask a few questions. I then called my regular vet and talked to the owner about their interest in developing a rehab program there. We met and decided that we would do that. I went to the course and realized that it was so much like human practice that I could begin right away. So, I began seeing dogs at Huron Animal Hospital in November 2002.

The big decision
At the end of December, I felt that I had to close down my small human private practice (it wasn't full time, but very lucrative); but wasn't sure why or what I would do. I gave my months' notice to the landlord and closed down at the end of January 2003, still wondering what would come up. I was working part-time doing home care, but that was it. Three days after I closed my office, Carrie emailed me and offered me a part time position as a

vet assistant at Alameda East Veterinary Hospital. Over the next couple of years, I gradually increased hours to three days a week and worked the other two days at a human outpatient orthopedic clinic. I became full time when Carrie left to work on her PhD at CSU at the end of August 2008.

A year later, the management at Alameda insisted that I go contract on a straight percentage because of legal issues and changes in our practice act. That's when I formed The K9 Body Shop, PC; however, I wasn't allowed to market myself as a separate business at Alameda East. I was contract there for another year-and-a-half and was doing some marketing and work with the DVMs (Doctor of Veterinary Medicine) in the Summit County (where many of the ski areas are). The administration at Alameda East then decided they wanted me to close down my business and become a salaried employee again. At that point, after spending so much energy, time and money in starting up my business, I knew I wouldn't be happy as an employee of a huge company anymore (Alameda East had been bought by VCA three years earlier). So, after working there for seven-and-a-half years, I left.

A new beginning!
I looked for space and started working part time in a suburb of Denver with a DVM who had a new underwater treadmill and nobody qualified to do rehab. That lasted seven months while I found a permanent location west of Denver in the location I'm in now. I moved into this location in December 2010. It's 35 minutes away from the other locations, so it has taken time to get to know some of the local vets and develop a new rapport. It has also taken time to build a patient load from a small following since I moved so far away from the other locations. But, in the long run, I believe that it was the right move and will pay off.

Even though the first two years here have been difficult, I'm seeing very slow, but consistent growth. I look forward to what lies ahead!

Tammy's business

Since my business is an out-patient office (independent of a veterinary hospital or clinic), I generally see about 65 cases per week. I also work alone with a part-time administrative assistant, so the patient load is gradually increasing as I get to know the DVMs in the area and more people are aware of where I am.

I have a pool, underwater treadmill, exercise balls and balance equipment, along with ultrasound, cold laser, and electrical stimulation available. I do a lot of manual therapy and have added dry needling, and I probably use manual techniques on 85% or more of the rehab dogs at some point in their therapy. Most dogs also get hydro at some point in their rehab. I use modalities infrequently, and I teach the owners to do most of the exercises at home.

The breakdown of cases I see is about; 70% ortho, 10% neuro, and 20% conditioning. Of these, approximately 25% are geriatric and the other ortho cases are split equally between acute/soft tissue injuries and post-op.

I charge by time and by the degree of technical skills needed for the treatment. For example, manual therapy is more expensive than a pool-swim of equal time. I have packages that are 10% off if a client wants to pay for ten visits ahead of time. I also have multi-dog discounts and discounts for working dogs (Police, seeing-eye dogs, etc.) and rescues who have dogs needing therapy before the dog is adopted. My initial consultation with treatment is an hour. Most other visits are 30 minutes, except I do have a small 15-minute charge for underwater treadmill.

As far as referrals go, about 50% of them come from DVMs and about 35% come from clients or former clients. The remaining 15% come from people surfing the internet or from other advertising I've done.

Getting the word out

I'm still experimenting with advertising and haven't found anything that consistently works other than word-of-mouth referrals from clients. I've found that going to canine events and setting up a tent is very expensive, time consuming and definitely does not work; I still do it occasionally, just to make sure. I do sponsor some athletic events, golf holes on golf courses, and go to local dog events unofficially and talk to people and hand out a few cards. This has seemed to be marginally effective. However, consistently giving excellent care and having clients refer their friend has been the least expensive and most productive marketing I've done. I'm also advertising in a canine magazine and DVM quarterly newsletter, both of which have been marginally effective.

The failure of some

Lack of public awareness of the profession is a big reason some fail. Plus, lack of awareness of the profession with the DVMs and their lack of willingness to change *"what they've always done."* It also has to do with DVMs who are not trained in physical therapy, claiming that they do physical therapy and doing it poorly, giving the whole specialty a bad name.

I also think the poor economy is a huge factor right now. In a good economy, I used to see dogs bi-weekly almost always. Now most people can only afford once-a-week visits or less.

My advice for those starting out: have a lot of extra cash to live on while the business is growing and expect the unexpected. Also, don't expect it to grow very fast. It will be at least two years until you will be able to live on what you make. Starting part-time is the best, if you can, by supplementing with other reliable work. Be patient with marketing. You won't see the returns the people you market to will promise when you meet with them.

How Tammy sees herself
I have a charming personality...
Seriously, people like to see you touching their dogs and the dogs responding with obvious relief. The personal, skillful touch that makes an immediate difference the owners can see is huge.

My Feldenkrais certification and training has made an immeasurable difference in how I practice and the results I get. I've used the theory and skills learned during that certification and combined it with the techniques I've learned in PT and by experience to get amazing results at times when it surprises me and the clients. That training in holistic movement, I think, is what we should have been taught in PT school.

I also try to find continuing education courses that I can apply to the animal world, (both PT courses and Feldenkrais courses). I practice on my patients and make up techniques as I go and remember the ones that are really effective and develop from there. I try to attend the CSM course to get feedback on what others are doing. I teach my new techniques, because teaching something always deepens your own understanding of what and why you are doing what you do. Until I started teaching final year PT students, I didn't realize that I had actually developed a new technique. It's been good for me to have to explain it and teach others to develop it further.

But there lies a problem

I believe the advanced training is greatly lacking for those of us who have been practicing for several years. I think we, as "old-timers," need to be writing and teaching more to help develop the profession and develop ourselves. However, as you know, it's difficult finding the time to do it or the resources, facility, etc. and to organize the teaching.

I'd like to do more writing (but I'm not sure who would publish it). I'd also like to look for publishing opportunities and teaching opportunities and continue with a long-term research project I'm doing.

Tammy's final thoughts

I think the opportunities will grow as more of the public becomes aware of Canine Rehab. It will be the public putting pressure on the DVM's that will get the job done, not the other way around.

Tania Costa,

CCRP, VT, CAAP, CMT
Canine Wellness Centre Inc
19 Waterman Ave, Unit 8,
Toronto, Ontario, Canada
www.caninewellness.com - 416-690-1077
E-mail: Tania@caninewellness.com

How did you get started, Tania?

At the age of 13, I thought I wanted to be a veterinarian, but after working at a vet clinic I realized that surgery and euthanasia were not aspects of the job I could deal with. Following various career paths, I ended up doing a degree in Interior Design. I worked in that field for 12 years, but in my time off I completed a certification in animal massage. Initially, I started training in canine massage for my own dogs. However, after I finished certification, I realized there was so much more to this field, and it was something I loved. So following the death of my mother in 2001, I decided that I needed to follow my passion—dogs! I received training first in the UK in the area of hydrotherapy (2002) before I realized that there was training in the USA for animal rehab. In 2002, I went back to school (while working part-time as a veterinary technician) to complete a diploma as a Veterinary Technician. This was a two-year process, and along the way I learned about the training program in animal rehab at the University of Tennessee. I enrolled in 2003. I completed the training in animal rehab and loved learning about the different ways I could help animals. In 2004 I started Canine Wellness Centre Inc., which at the time was a huge undertaking. I visited several vet clinics in the Toronto area, telling veterinarians about what I wanted to do. In most cases I was told, "This will never fly!" With determination, I forged ahead, believing this was something that was needed in the Toronto area.

I remember my first patient, a dog with a TPLO. I was scared out of my mind about how to do PROM and use my ultrasound machine. Today, I laugh at that memory! It was scary, but I studied all my notes, reviewed videos from class and did what I was trained to do. The dog did great and today (still is a client of mine after yet another TPLO and now arthritis) he is still benefiting from rehabilitation.

In 2007, I realized that I needed yet another tool to provide a wider range of rehabilitation techniques. I enrolled in Tallgrass Animal Acupressure Institute, to learn about TCM and animal acupressure. To this date I use this for pain management and for providing further rehabilitation modalities for helping dogs that come to my facility. I am now a certified assistant-trainer at Tallgrass Animal Acupressure Institute, and I use the skills I learned there with many of the animals I work with. In 2009, I furthered my training with Patricia Kortekaas of Full Spectrum Canine Therapy (www.fullspectrumcaninetherapy.com) to learn more hands-on techniques for helping the dogs I treat. Now, as of 2011, I have completed all levels of osteopathy and use this in 50% of my caseload.

As you can see, the area of rehabilitation is an area that has so many different offerings. To be the best practitioner you need to constantly upgrade your skills and obtain continued training to provide the best possible solution for the clients that you work with.

Tell us more about your practice

My facility is 3200 square feet; it has a rehab area for exercises, treatment area, and a rehab pool (16' X 7') with underwater treadmill. We now provide a second pool (20' X 7') for recovered patients, those with minor arthritis, for weight loss, and for those just looking for a fun and safe swimming experience in the winter months.

Additionally, we provide wheelchair fittings, weight loss pro-grams (woof watchers), grooming for disabled dogs, seminars on core conditioning for athletic dogs, as well as an in-house pros-thetic/orthotist for dogs that require products for supporting joints that cannot undergo surgery. I also make assistive devices (slings, ortho beds, icers, etc. for dogs that require assistance), and we have a referral network of certified veterinary acupunc-turists and chiropractors.

We see about 50-60 rehab cases per week, and 15 – 20 recrea-tional swimmers per week. The caseload breaks down to be 55% orthopaedic, 20% neurologic, 20% geriatric, and 5% fitness or weight loss. Staffing consists of myself plus two veterinary assis-tants, one who is currently learning rehab. All of my patients are referrals from local (within 40km) veterinarians.

A typical rehab session includes the following: First I check the dog over to see how the joint or issue is progressing (assess-ment), then I review exercises for home use with the owner and have them perform them with me. Following this, I perform a modality that is warranted (laser, ultrasound, E-stim, osteopa-thy, massage, etc.). If the case warrants, we end with an under-water treadmill (UWTM) session or in neuro cases, we use the land treadmill for gait retraining. We try water, but if the legs do not move in water, the land treadmill is utilized.

We tend to bill by the service.

Rehab is for a 30-40 minute session (includes whatever modality/manual therapy/UWTM that is required)

Wellness is for just UWTM sessions

Massage (30 or 60 minutes)

Acupressure (60 minutes)

Osteopathy (60 minutes)

Recreational swimming (20 or 30 minute sessions)

Weight loss counseling

We do not charge for each different modality (equipment), so a rehab session would include whatever is needed to do the job properly.

What about getting referrals and advertising?

Patients access my services by veterinary referral only; however, in many cases, they hear about me through dog walkers, past clients, or veterinary technicians. When they call, they are told they must get a referral from their veterinarian. I find that once the veterinarian sees changes, he/she becomes a "bought-in" referral source and continues to send clients directly. Also, I get several referrals from local ortho/neuro specialty referral centers that have included me on their listing of rehabilitation practitioners.

The only advertising I do is in a local dog newspaper. I have found advertising in vet magazines and newspapers does not have a return on investment. The best advertising is word of mouth and educating veterinarians. I have advertised in local veterinary association magazines, which has yielded NO return on investment! I also offer free one-time sessions for veterinarians and veterinary technicians to bring their dog and experience what rehab is about and see the benefits.

Why do you think you have been successful?

I have spent time to learn manual skills as well as the basic canine rehabilitation education. Each dog I work with is provided an initial assessment. During the assessment, I evaluate the dog's condition and diagnosis, viability of the different modalities that I provide, and discuss the client's goals. Typically, within a session, I will combine osteopathy, traditional Chinese medicine (TCM) and massage, as well as laser therapy and land exercises. With 60% of cases, they finish a session in the UWTM. At each session I evaluate the patient, discuss the past week, and review exercises to determine an appropriate treatment protocol for that specific day.

An important strength, however, is empowering owners with helping their pets and educating vets about what I do in order to help their clients. Continued support is important as well.

I take many calls from clients before they even go to their vet! Sometimes, I simply coach them on what to discuss with their vet. There are times when a dog is referred for a particular diagnosis and I find some other problems. In those instances, the dog is immediately (and diplomatically) sent back to the referring veterinarian for further testing. I also have many vets that call me to review a case to see if I can figure out what is going on. Some will admit that they do not remember (or did not learn) certain tests or diagnostics for addressing some orthopaedic issues. In summary, I think that both the veterinarians and my clients have learned that I continue my passion and learning in this area, and that I support both the client and the referring veterinarian to make the overall case more successful.

What has been your greatest struggle or challenge in practice?

Dealing with veterinarians who feel that rehabilitation is the "last line" of treatment has been aggravating. Mostly they have learned to refer clients following TPLO or hip surgeries, but other cases still get left behind. It can be frustrating when you have a dog come in with severe chronic pain from osteoarthritis. Medication is not providing enough pain relief, and the owners are looking for more options. Some veterinarians seem to think of rehabilitation as a last resort instead of a two-tiered, complementary treatment regime. I have also had some cases of dogs being paralyzed following IVDD surgery; they did not walk following surgery. Neurologists often tell owners there is no hope despite it being only three weeks later—but the clients have spent thousands of dollars and want their beloved pet to walk again. In many instances, with proper re-education, laser, and gait retraining, these dogs can lead a life of walking without a wheelchair. In each of these cases the owner is cautioned that walking may not be achievable, but in an ideal world, it be great if owners were at least given the information about all the treatment options available!

What about the rehab facilities, departments, or practitioners that fail?

This is a hard one. There are only a few near me, but from what I can see (as I tend to see patients from these facilities) is that they seem to think that the UWTM is the "be-all-and-end-all" in rehab. They have a paralyzed dog, they put him in the water... but if he does not move his legs, well then, rehab won't work! So I guess what this says is that my competitors do not have the manual skills to provide a higher level of rehabilitation therapy. I also think that my competitors do not engage in continued training in rehab. So they only have the initial skills learned in school, but since the rehab world is constantly expanding, they are not providing current rehab skills.

What do you think about the educational opportunities in the field of canine rehabilitation?
From my experience (I trained at Tennessee), the University of Tennessee canine rehab program is strong in scientific evidence, but lacks in hands-on. This is why I completed additional training in these areas. I have tried on several occasions to do training at the Canine Rehabilitation Institute (for the hands-on training), but they will only do this if you (as a technician) have a veterinarian that will basically support and oversee you. They will not look at your experience or outside skill levels. This does not allow for those who want to further their education to learn more and expand the field.

In my mind what would be great is a school that provides both manual training and scientific evidence (and not Dr. Millis talking about his thousands of knee surgeries!) When we get out in the field, we must have clients understand what surgery they had or will have, what it means, and how it will impact their dog's life. An owner that has all the information can make an informed decision. I always thoroughly educate my clients, as I want them to understand what their dog has gone through (even if it is arthritis) and what it means in the long term. Knowledge is power... a mantra I live by.

I also think schools should broaden their horizons and provide other types of "continuing education" to ensure students have been exposed to everything rehabilitation has to offer (i.e. wheelchair fittings, osteopathy, massage, advanced physiotherapy techniques, hospice care, etc.).

I go to most all conferences, training, and symposiums in the area of rehabilitation and complementary health care. I feel this is necessary for this growing field—to learn from others and share ideas on how to help our patients.

What is your next step as an animal rehabilitation practitioner?

I plan to continue to seek out more training courses, expanding my business to having another rehab practitioner to assist in caseload management, and acquiring a veterinarian on the premises. (Currently, I am not allowed to have a DVM or PT on the premises due to College of Veterinarians of Ontario guidelines.)

Would you have done anything differently?

I would not have got myself so much in debt! I would have bought different modalities in a staggered fashion as needs presented. The biggest thing, however, I would have designed my pools completely differently. Unfortunately, at the time there were no doggie pools available for me to model after or learn from! (These were very costly mistakes!)

Future vision and advice...

I would like to see the field expand to include acceptance of veterinarians, physical therapists and veterinary technicians as valued members of this growing field. If I was able, I would have a physical therapist on staff, as well as a veterinarian, to be able to provide continued support, shared experience and better care for clients. I would also love to see more continuing education courses with experts in the field to be able to share their knowledge and expertise.

My advice to rehab practitioners getting started is to understand the huge investment of money, time and commitment to continued training despite trying to run a business. To grow a business, owners have to look at the bottom line, pay bills, maximize time and space. To be more successful it is also important to look at your demographics and to provide secondary/tertiary services to exceed client expectations.

Made in the USA
San Bernardino, CA
10 March 2014